Healthy Brain Aging: Evidence Based Methods to Preserve Brain Function and Prevent Dementia

Guest Editor

ABHILASH K. DESAI, MD, FAPA

CLINICS IN GERIATRIC MEDICINE

www.geriatric.theclinics.com

February 2010 • Volume 26 • Number 1

SAUNDERS an imprint of ELSEVIER, Inc.

W.B. SAUNDERS COMPANY
A Division of Elsevier Inc.

1600 John F. Kennedy Blvd., Suite 1800. Philadelphia, Pennsylvania 19103-2899

http://www.theclinics.com

CLINICS IN GERIATRIC MEDICINE Volume 26, Number 1
February 2010 ISSN 0749–0690, ISBN-13: 978-1-4377-1822-5

Editor: Yonah Korngold

Clinics in Geriatric Medicine (ISSN 0749-0690) is published quarterly by Elsevier Inc., 360 Park Avenue South, New York, NY 10010-1710. Months of issue are February, May, August, and November. Business and Editorial Offices: 1600 John F. Kennedy Blvd., Suite 1800, Philadelphia, PA 191023-2899. Periodicals postage paid at New York, NY, and additional mailing offices. Subscription prices is $225.00 per year (US individuals), $388.00 per year (US institutions), $293.00 per year (Canadian individuals), $484.00 per year (Canadian institutions), $311.00 per year (foreign individuals) and $484.00 per year (foreign institutions). Foreign air speed delivery is included in all *Clinics* subscription prices. All prices are subject to change without notice. POSTMASTER: Send address changes to *Clinics in Geriatric Medicine,* Elsevier Health Sciences Division, Subscription Customer Service, 3251 Riverport Lane, Maryland Heights, MO 63043. Telephone: 1-800-654-2452 (U.S. and Canada); 314-447-8871 (outside U.S. and Canada). Fax: 314-447-8029. E-mail: journalscustomerservice-usa@elsevier.com (for print support) or journalsonlinesupport-usa@elsevier.com (for online support).

Reprints. For copies of 100 or more, of articles in this publication, please contact the Commercial Reprints Department, Elsevier Inc., 360 Park Avenue South, New York, New York 10010-1710. Tel.: (212) 633-3812; Fax: (212) 462-1935, email: reprints@elsevier.com.

Clinics in Geriatric Medicine is covered in *MEDLINE/PubMed (Index Medicus), EMBASE/Excerpta Medica, Current Contents/Clinical Medicine (CC/CM), and the Cumulative Index to Nursing & Allied Health Literature.*

Printed in the United States of America.

Contributors

GUEST EDITOR

ABHILASH K. DESAI, MD, FAPA
Associate Professor, Director, Center for Healthy Brain Aging, Department of Neurology and Psychiatry, Division of Geriatric Psychiatry; Associate Professor, Department of Internal Medicine, Division of Geriatric Medicine, Saint Louis University School of Medicine, St Louis, Missouri

AUTHORS

GABOR ABELLAN VAN KAN, MD
Department of Geriatric Medicine, CHU Toulouse; Geriatrician, Service de Médecine Interne et de Gérontologie Clinique, Pavillon Junod, Hôpital La Grave-Casselardit, Toulouse, France

NAZEM BASSIL, MD
Department of Neurology and Psychiatry, Division of Geriatric Psychiatry, Saint Louis University, St Louis, Missouri

ANNE D. BASTING, PhD
Director of the Center on Age and Community; Associate Professor of Theatre, University of Wisconsin Milwaukee, Milwaukee, Wisconsin

JOHN T. CHIBNALL, PhD
Professor, Department of Neurology and Psychiatry, Saint Louis University School of Medicine, St Louis, Missouri

ABHILASH K. DESAI, MD, FAPA
Associate Professor, Director, Center for Healthy Brain Aging, Department of Neurology and Psychiatry, Division of Geriatric Psychiatry; Associate Professor, Department of Internal Medicine, Division of Geriatric Medicine, Saint Louis University School of Medicine, St Louis, Missouri

LEON FLICKER, MB BS, PhD, FRACP
Director, Western Australian Centre for Health and Ageing, CMR, Western Australian Institute for Medical Research; Professor of Geriatric Medicine, School of Medicine and Pharmacology, University of Western Australia, Perth, Australia

JAMES E. GALVIN, MD, MPH
Associate Professor, Alzheimer Disease Research Center; Department of Neurology; Department of Psychiatry; Department of Neurobiology, Washington University School of Medicine, St Louis, Missouri

GEORGE T. GROSSBERG, MD
Samuel W. Fordyce Professor, Director, Division of Geriatric Psychiatry, Department of Neurology and Psychiatry, Saint Louis University School of Medicine, St Louis, Missouri

ANJALI S. KAMAT, MD
Geriatric Medicine Fellow, Division of Geriatric Medicine, Department of Internal Medicine, Saint Louis University School of Medicine, St Louis, Missouri

SANJEEV M. KAMAT, MD
Staff Psychiatrist, Department of Psychiatry, St Alexius Hospital and Forest Park Hospital, St Louis, Missouri; Department of Psychiatry, Jefferson Regional Medical Center, Crystal City, Missouri; Voluntary Faculty, Department of Neurology and Psychiatry, Saint Louis University School of Medicine, St Louis, Missouri

LAURENCE J. KINSELLA, MD, FAAN
Professor of Neurology and Psychiatry, Saint Louis University; Chief, Neurology and Neurophysiology, Forest Park Hospital, St Louis, Missouri

VIKAS KUMAR, MD, PhD
Chief Resident, Department of Neurology and Psychiatry, Saint Louis University, St Louis, Missouri

ASENATH LA RUE, PhD
Senior Scientist, Wisconsin Alzheimer's Institute, School of Medicine and Public Health, University of Wisconsin – Madison, Madison, Wisconsin

RAMAN K. MALHOTRA, MD
Co-Director, SLUCare Sleep Disorders Center; Assistant Professor, Department of Neurology and Psychiatry, Saint Louis University School of Medicine, St Louis, Missouri

SUSAN H. MCFADDEN, PhD
Professor of Psychology, Department of Psychology, University of Wisconsin Oshkosh, Oshkosh, Wisconsin

JOHN E. MORLEY, MB, BCh
Department of Internal Medicine, Division of Geriatric Medicine, Saint Louis University School of Medicine; Geriatric Research Education and Clinical Center, Veterans Affairs Medical Center, St Louis, Missouri

YVES ROLLAND, MD, PhD
Inserm; University of Toulouse III; Professor of Geriatrics, Department of Geriatric Medicine, CHU Toulouse; Service de Médecine Interne et de Gérontologie Clinique, Pavillon Junod, Hôpital La Grave-Casselardit, Toulouse, France

RAWAN TARAWNEH, MD
Fellow, Alzheimer Disease Research Center; Department of Neurology, Washington University School of Medicine, St Louis, Missouri

BRUNO VELLAS, MD, PhD
Inserm; University of Toulouse III; Professor of Geriatrics, Department of Geriatric Medicine, CHU Toulouse; Service de Médecine Interne et de Gérontologie Clinique, Pavillon Junod, Hôpital La Grave-Casselardit, Toulouse, France

Contents

> Optimal cognitive function is vital to independence, productivity, and quality of life, and the debilitation associated with dementias makes them the most feared of conditions related to aging. Effective preventive measures are key components of any response to the potentially overwhelming problem of dementias. Increasing evidence points to the potential risk roles of vascular factors and disorders (eg, midlife obesity, dyslipidemia, diabetes, high blood pressure, cigarette smoking, and cerebrovascular lesions) and the potential protective roles of psychosocial factors (eg, higher education, regular exercise, healthy diet, intellectually challenging leisure activities, and active socially integrated lifestyle) in the pathogenic process and clinical manifestation of dementing disorders. Optimal control of vascular risk factors, secondary prevention of stroke, and manipulation of lifestyle factors have demonstrated efficacy in prevention of stroke and myocardial infarction. Thus, adding dementia prevention and brain function preservation as goals to already existing or planned prevention efforts is appropriate and necessary. Age must be taken into account when assessing the likely effect of such interventions against dementia, which underscores the need to begin prevention efforts early in patients' lives.

> Cardiovascular risk factors have been associated with 2 common manifestation of unhealthy brain in older people, cognitive impairment and depression. The evidence for these effects is almost entirely observational, but links hypertension, smoking, hypercholesterolemia, diabetes mellitus, and hyperhomocysteinemia with cognitive impairment and depression. Unfortunately randomized trials evaluating interventions for these risk factors on the outcomes of cognition or mood have either been inconclusive or negative. However, as there are considerable other health benefits from targeting cardiovascular risk factors, these interventions should be more widely adopted, which would also probably result in positive outcomes for the brain.

> Head injury has been recognized as an increasingly important determinant of late-life cognitive function. Despite a large number of research and clinical studies, no direct link has been established between minor head

trauma with or without loss of consciousness and the development of dementia of the Alzheimer type. Similarly for alcohol, low doses have been found to be somewhat protective against dementia, whereas large doses increased the risk of late-life cognitive dysfunction. Among the many environmental toxins suspected of causing cognitive dysfunction, lead intoxication has the strongest evidence to support a link.

Sleep plays an important role in learning, memory encoding, and cognition. Insufficient quantity or quality of sleep leads not only to short-term neurocognitive dysfunction but also to permanent changes to the central nervous system. Sleep disorders are common in the geriatric population. The hypoxemia and sleep fragmentation resulting from obstructive sleep apnea are the most likely pathophysiology responsible for damage to the brain. Because treatment of these sleep disorders can lead to improved cognitive function, it is becoming increasingly important for physicians to be able to correctly recognize and treat these disorders in patients presenting with memory or cognitive complaints.

There is a long history of hormones altering behavior and endocrinopathies playing a role in psychiatric disease. This article highlights the hormonal changes that occur with aging and the effects of these hormonal changes on the brain, concentrating not on the well-known psychiatric manifestations of endocrine diseases, but on the more subtle effects of hormones and metabolic alteration seen in many older persons. The article focuses predominately on the role of hormones in cognition, as dementia and mild cognitive impairment are major problems in the older individual.

There is increasing evidence to suggest that physical activity has a protective effect on brain functioning in older people. To date, no randomized controlled trial (RCT) has shown that regular physical activity prevents dementia, but recent RCTs suggests an improvement of cognitive functioning in persons involved in aerobic programs, and evidence is accumulating from basic research. Future prevention of Alzheimer disease may depend on lifestyle habits such as physical activity.

Severe nutritional deficiencies, such as protein energy malnutrition and deficiency of nicotinamide, vitamin B_{12}, folate, and thiamine, have long been recognized to cause severe confusion. Lesser vitamin deficiencies have been linked to the pathogenesis of delirium. Hypo- and hyperglycemia and hypertriglyceridemia can cause cognitive deficits. Epidemiologic and animal studies have linked several other nutrients (omega-3 fatty acids, lutein, alpha-lipoic acid, and the Mediterranean diet) to cognitive performance and the prevention of dementia.

Current knowledge about the roles of cognitively stimulating lifestyles and cognitive training interventions in preserving cognitive function in later life is reviewed. Potential mechanisms for beneficial effects of cognitive stimulation and training are discussed, and key gaps in research identified. Suggestions are provided for advising patients about brain-healthy lifestyles, acknowledging that much remains to be learned in this area of research. More randomized controlled trials, using challenging regimes of training and stimulation and long-term follow-up, are needed, measuring cognitive trajectories in normal aging and relative risk of Alzheimer disease as outcomes.

The term dementia refers to memory impairment and loss of other intellectual abilities, which interfere with normal daily activities. Alzheimer disease is a type of dementia that accounts for 50% to 70% of dementia cases. Although the precise reason behind dementia is unknown, there are several risk factors that increase the risk for the development for dementia and several protective factors that may protect against the development of dementia. This article reviews potential risk factors and protective factors for the development of dementia, and in particular Alzheimer disease, and discusses the challenges in developing a dementia risk index.

The cellular mechanisms underlying neuronal loss and neurodegeneration have been an area of interest in the last decade. Although neurodegenerative diseases such as Alzheimer disease, Parkinson disease, and Huntington disease each have distinct clinical symptoms and pathologies, they all share common mechanisms such as protein aggregation, oxidative injury, inflammation, apoptosis, and mitochondrial injury that contribute to neuronal loss. Although cerebrovascular disease has different causes from the neurodegenerative disorders, many of the same common disease mechanisms come into play following a stroke. Novel therapies that target each of these mechanisms may be effective in decreasing the risk of disease, abating symptoms, or slowing down their progression. Although most of these therapies are experimental, and require further investigation, a few seem to offer promise.

Susan H. McFadden and Anne D. Basting

Creative engagement, as an expression of and a support for resilience, may have a neuroprotective effect among older adults, contributing to retention of cognitive capacity. Recent research on creative activities shows that they strengthen social networks and give persons a sense of control; both outcomes have been associated with brain health. The authors cite evidence suggesting that positive social interactions can nurture resilience and creative engagement among older persons, including those living with dementia. The motivational, attentional, affective, and social components of creative activities combine to offer older persons meaningful opportunities to express and strengthen their resilience, regardless of their cognitive status, despite the biopsychosocial challenges of aging. The article addresses implications for future research, clinical practice, and public policy, and suggests how gaps in current research on resilience and creativity might be addressed.

THE CLINICS ARE NOW AVAILABLE ONLINE!

Access your subscription at:
www.theclinics.com

Preface

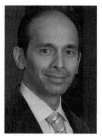

Abhilash K. Desai, MD, FAPA
Guest Editor

This special issue of *Clinics in Geriatric Medicine*: "Healthy Brain Aging: Evidence Based Methods to Preserve Brain Function and Prevent Dementia," is devoted to cognitive health, a major factor in ensuring good quality of life and preserving independence in middle aged and older adults. As the readers of *Clinics in Geriatric Medicine* are well aware, the United States population as a whole is aging at an unprecedented rate. With that comes an increasing incidence of disabling cognitive decline due to a variety of conditions (especially Alzheimer disease and other dementias). The articles in this special issue describe the results of research in the last 2 decades regarding risk and protective factors for late-life cognitive decline and potential implications of these results on clinical care, public education, future research, and public policy. These articles provide important support for evidence-based strategies to preserve brain function and prevent dementias (especially Alzheimer disease and vascular cognitive impairment), strategies that can be implemented in clinical practice and that future research can further improve upon. A significant attribute of this special issue is the diversity of expertise of authors from the United States, Europe, and Australia, including geriatric psychiatrists, geriatricians, neurologists, neuropsychologists, and psychologists.

I hope that the research presented in this special issue will improve our ability to disseminate effective cognitive health messages. Furthermore, I am optimistic that these data will contribute to the development of interventions that generate action in local communities and eventually result in improved public health.

This special issue is an invitation to every clinician, individual, and family to make healthy brain aging a priority. The findings presented here fit into a larger and

Clin Geriatr Med 26 (2010) xi–xii
doi:10.1016/j.cger.2009.12.007   **geriatric.theclinics.com**

burgeoning view of prevention of late-life cognitive impairment through application, at least by midlife, of as many healthy behaviors as possible.

Abhilash K. Desai, MD, FAPA
Center for Healthy Brain Aging
Department of Neurology and Psychiatry
Division of Geriatric Psychiatry
and
Department of Internal Medicine
Division of Geriatric Medicine
Saint Louis University School of Medicine
1438 South Grand Boulevard
St Louis, MO 63104, USA

E-mail address:
adesai@slu.edu

Healthy Brain Aging: A Road Map

Abhilash K. Desai, MD[a,b,]*, George T. Grossberg, MD[a],
John T. Chibnall, PhD[c]

KEYWORDS

- Dementia • Prevention • Healthy • Brain
- Aging • Cognition • Alzheimer's disease
- Vascular cognitive impairment

With the rapidly growing number of elderly individuals at risk for cognitive decline, finding ways to maintain or improve cognitive health and quality of life for this population has become a public health priority.[1,2,3,4] Many middle-aged and older adults worry that a memory slip may be an early sign of Alzheimer disease (AD). Moreover, they are also asking physicians what they can do to maintain cognitive vitality and preserve their memory as they age. Regardless of gender, race, ethnicity, language, or geographic region, older adults have indicated that cognitive function (memory, decision-making, and similar functions) is important to healthy aging.[4,5] Modification of risk factors remains a cornerstone for dementia prevention until disease-modifying agents prove efficacious. Moderately strong evidence indicates that lifestyle factors, vascular risk factors (VRFs), and cerebrovascular disease are major factors in the pathogenesis of dementia, particularly AD and vascular cognitive impairment (VCI).[6,7] The evidence that lifestyle and VRFs have reduced the rates of myocardial infarction and stroke is strong. Therefore, targeting these risk factors for the prevention of dementia is also appropriate.[6–8] This constitutes risk factors to avoid (eg, obesity, dyslipidemia, diabetes, high blood pressure, cigarette smoking). On the other hand, health professionals should educate patients, especially patients at higher risk of AD and VCI, about proactive strategies that may increase the odds of healthier aging. This constitutes protective factors to embrace (eg, challenging the brain intellectually, exercise, proper diet, active socially integrated lifestyle). Despite growing evidence of these modifiable risk and protective factors for future dementia, there is continued lack of

Disclosures: None.

[a] Department of Neurology and Psychiatry, Division of Geriatric Psychiatry, Saint Louis University School of Medicine, 1438 South Grand Boulevard, St Louis, MO 63104, USA

[b] Department of Internal Medicine, Division of Geriatric Medicine, Saint Louis University School of Medicine, 1438 South Grand Boulevard, St Louis, MO 63104, USA

[c] Department of Neurology and Psychiatry, Saint Louis University School of Medicine, 1438 South Grand Boulevard, St Louis, MO 63104, USA

* Corresponding author. Department of Neurology and Psychiatry, Division of Geriatric Psychiatry, Saint Louis University, 1438 South Grand Boulevard, St Louis, MO 63104.

E-mail address: adesai@slu.edu (A.K. Desai).

Clin Geriatr Med 26 (2010) 1–16

doi:10.1016/j.cger.2009.12.002

geriatric.theclinics.com

awareness among lay people and health care professionals alike about evidence-based strategies to maintain cognitive health.[1] This article provides a road map to implement these multidomain interventions toward preserving brain function and reducing risks for future dementia. The road map for a healthy aging brain involves 9 steps, as outlined in **Table 1**.

STEP 1: UNDERSTANDING THE DEMOGRAPHIC IMPERATIVE

Dementia is characterized by a loss of or decline in cognitive abilities (eg, memory, language), accompanied by significant decline in daily functioning and change in behavior. Degenerative dementias include AD, Parkinson disease dementia (PDD), dementia with Lewy bodies (DLB), and frontotemporal dementias (FTDs). VCI encompasses several syndromes: vascular dementia (including poststroke and multi-infarct dementia); mixed primary neurodegenerative disease and vascular dementia; and cognitive impairment of vascular origin that does not meet dementia criteria.[9] Together, these dementias account for more than 90% of all dementias in older adults. They are all progressive and irreversible. There are no definitive treatments to halt or slow the relentless cognitive decline that accompanies these dementias, although the long-term course of decline is highly variable in different patients and in the same patient over time. Growing neuropathologic evidence indicates that most dementias have neurodegenerative (most commonly AD) and vascular features and these seem to act synergistically.[10]

Mild cognitive impairment (MCI) is a condition in which the individual has cognitive decline that is severe enough to be noticeable to others and that shows up on cognitive tests, but is not severe enough to interfere with daily life. There is increasing evidence that MCI defines a group of persons who are at near-term risk of developing dementia and particularly AD.[11]

After the reproductive years, evolution has not provided a great deal of protection for enhanced survival.[12] As a result, aging produces a permissible environment, allowing opportunistic disease processes to develop, including cerebrovascular disease, AD, PDD, DLB, and the FTDs. The incidence and prevalence of dementia are expected to increase several-fold in the coming decades. Population epidemiologic studies of

Table 1	
Nine steps to healthy brain aging	
Step 1	Understanding the demographic imperative
Step 2	Understanding the concept of healthy brain aging
Step 3	Understanding that prevention of dementia primarily involves delaying onset of dementia
Step 4	Understanding the various evidence-based strategies to promote healthy brain aging
Step 5	Understanding who the target population is, when to start applying these interventions, and when to stop
Step 6	Understanding the potential for brain changes (neuroplasticity), the capacity of the brain to generate new brain cells (neurogenesis), and the concept of CR
Step 7	Understanding the directions that future research needs to take to make healthy brain aging a reality for all
Step 8	Understanding the role of government, health-insurance companies, and academic institutions in promoting healthy brain aging
Step 9	Understanding the role of physicians and individuals in promoting healthy brain aging

dementia have revealed a steady increase in the incidence of dementia into old age.[13] With average life expectancy in the United States approaching 80 years, the greatest demographic change is the increasing number of persons more than 85 years of age, in whom most cases of dementia occur. Currently, an estimated 5.3 million Americans are affected by AD and other dementias.[13] In the coming decades, the baby boom population is projected to add 10 million people to these numbers. Further, as many as 10% to 20% of people aged 65 years and older have MCI.[13] There are 78 million baby boomers currently and a substantial proportion of them have multiple cardiovascular risk factors. Thus, the total population at risk for future dementia is high and this constitutes the demographic imperative.

STEP 2: UNDERSTANDING THE CONCEPT OF HEALTHY BRAIN AGING

Components of healthy cognitive functioning include language, thought, memory, executive function (ie, the ability to plan and carry out tasks), judgment, attention, perception, and ability to live a purposeful life. In 2005, the Critical Evaluation Study Committee was formed as part of the trans-National Institutes of Health (NIH; the National Institute on Aging, the National Institute of Mental Health, and the National Institute of Neurologic Disorders and Stroke) Project on Cognitive and Emotional Health. The definition of cognitive health adopted by the Critical Evaluation Study Committee was that cognitive health as it pertains to the older adult should be defined not just as the absence of disease but also as the development and preservation of the multidimensional cognitive structure that allows the older adult to maintain social connectedness, an ongoing sense of purpose, and the abilities to function independently, to recover functionally from illness or injury, and to cope with residual functional deficits.[2] This definition of "healthy cognitive aging" (synonymous with "healthy brain aging" for the purposes of this article) is more comprehensive and proactive than what is embraced by most clinicians, where healthy cognitive aging implies only a relative lack of cognitive decline with aging.

Dementia is not inevitable with aging, given the average life expectancy of most people. Neuropsychological and neuropathologic correlations suggest that there are centenarians (conservative estimate 20%) who demonstrate no evidence of cognitive decline or neurodegenerative disease.[14] Initial evidence suggests that most of the supercentenarians (at least 110 years old) markedly delay and even escape clinical expression of neurodegenerative diseases (AD, Parkinson disease) and cerebrovascular disease toward the end of their exceptionally long lives.[15,16] Prevalence of dementia was only 25% in the only population-based, prospective clinical study of supercentenarians.[16] Thus, centenarians and supercentenarians can be considered models for healthy brain aging for purposes of research, as studying them may reveal neurobiological mechanisms that play a protective role against neuropathologies involved in dementing disorders.

STEP 3: UNDERSTANDING THAT PREVENTION OF DEMENTIA PRIMARILY INVOLVES DELAYING ONSET OF DEMENTIA

Because the most common forms of dementia affect the old and very old, even a modest delay in the appearance or worsening of cognitive deterioration would translate into a large reduction in the incidence of disease (as these people would die from other causes before entering an overt stage of dementia). Indeed, it is estimated that among the 106 million cases of AD expected globally by the year 2050, about 23 million (or >20%) could be avoided completely if it were possible to delay the start of disease by 2 years, beginning in the year 2010.[17] An average 1-year delay in disease onset would result in annual savings of nearly $10 billion in 10 years.[18] Because AD and VCI account for more than 80% of dementias and research to date on risk and protective factors for dementia have primarily focused on AD and VCI, this discussion of cognitive decline focuses mainly on delaying the onset of AD and VCI.

Neurodegenerative disorders and atherosclerosis begin early in life and progress unnoticed for decades before they are clinically expressed.[19,20] Such a long process of development of AD and VCI provides great opportunity for instituting strategies to slow the pathogenic processes over several years with the hope that onset of dementia can be delayed.

STEP 4: UNDERSTANDING THE VARIOUS EVIDENCE-BASED STRATEGIES TO PROMOTE HEALTHY BRAIN AGING

Evidence-based strategies to promote healthy brain aging include lifestyle modification, optimal control of VRFs, secondary prevention of stroke, medications, and strategies to reduce psychological distress.

Lifestyle, VRFs, and Secondary Prevention of Stroke

Increasing evidence strongly points to the potential risk roles of VRFs and disorders (eg, midlife obesity, dyslipidemia, diabetes, high blood pressure, cigarette smoking, obstructive sleep apnea, and cerebrovascular lesions) and the potential protective roles of psychosocial factors (eg, higher education, regular exercise, healthy diet, intellectually challenging leisure activity, and active socially integrated lifestyle) in the pathogenic process and clinical manifestation of the dementing disorders (especially AD and VCI) (see the articles by Flicker; Kumar and Kinsella; McFadden and Basting; Kamat and colleagues; Morley and Bassil; La Rue; Rolland and colleagues; Malhotra and Desai; and Morley elsewhere in this issue).[6–8,21,22] Thus, promoting healthy lifestyle, optimal control of VRFs, and secondary prevention of stroke as potential strategies to reduce dementia risk are prudent, despite absence of evidence from randomized controlled trials (RCTs) of risk-factor modification (except for hypertension, for which the evidence is mixed). Integrative interventions (eg, exercise, healthy diet, medications) focusing on overall risk instead of individual risk factors may bring more benefit to individuals at risk.

Despite the existence of expert consensus guidelines on cardiovascular prevention by the American College of Cardiology and the American Heart Association, the implementation of risk-reduction practices for cardiovascular disease remains suboptimal.[23,24] For example, in a sample of 364 community-dwelling stroke survivors aged 34 to 88 years, more than 90% had at least 2 concurrent risk factors that were inadequately treated.[25] Among patients admitted to hospital with a stroke associated with atrial fibrillation, only 50% of ideal candidates for anticoagulation therapy were started on warfarin.[26] The proportion of individuals with hypertension achieving control of blood pressure was low (approximately 33%) in those without diabetes and very low (approximately 15%) in those with diabetes.[27] Only 3% of the population in the United States follows the 4 basic healthy habits: no smoking, 30 minutes of moderate intensity exercise 5 days a week, eating 5 servings of fruit and vegetables per day, and maintaining a normal body weight.[28]

Practical application of various strategies in patients' daily life can be promoted by use of a simple checklist (**Table 2**) developed by the authors and routinely used at the Center for Healthy Brain Aging, Saint Louis University School of Medicine, St Louis, MO, USA. These strategies when used in combination may have an additive effect.

Coexisting medical conditions, such as pulmonary disease, heart failure, renal insufficiency, drug-induced cognitive impairment, sleep apnea, vitamin deficiencies, depression, metabolic and endocrine disturbances, and the systemic effects of other failing organs can all negatively affect cognition.[29] Even in the presence of mild to moderate AD lesions or cerebrovascular lesions, these conditions may drive synaptic and neuronal loss, resulting in brain atrophy and dementia. Conversely, absence of these factors might allow a person to remain cognitively intact despite some accumulation of lesions caused by neurodegeneration and cerebrovascular disease. Thus, addressing these conditions is also important.

Medications to Prevent Dementia

No effective pharmacologic intervention has been found to prevent AD or other neurodegenerative dementias. There is insufficient evidence for the prescribing of medications such as acetylsalicylic acid, nonsteroidal antiinflammatory drugs, statins, vitamin E or C, and COX-2 inhibitors for the sole purpose of reducing the risk of dementia or MCI.[6,30,31] There is good evidence to avoid estrogens (alone or in combination with progesterone) and high-dose vitamin E (>400 IU/d) for the sole purpose of reducing dementia risk (see the article by Morley and Bassil elsewhere in this issue).[6] High-dose vitamin E (400 IU/d) was associated with increased risk of hemorrhagic stroke in a recent cardiovascular prevention study.[32] The authors recommend caution in using vitamins to prevent dementias because preliminary evidence suggests that antioxidants (eg, vitamins C and E) may reduce the health-promoting effects of exercise.[33] Physicians may choose to advise their patients about the advantages of daily omega-3 supplements and vitamin D on overall health and cardiovascular health, and potential benefits in promoting brain health (see the article by Morley elsewhere in this issue).[34] Physicians are encouraged to discuss the risks and benefits of various medications, vitamins, supplements, and herbal remedies for the promotion of overall health, including their potential effect on cognitive health. Several new therapies to limit the accumulation of amyloid deposits are in late-phase clinical trials and may become available within the next few years (see the article by Tarawneh and Galvin elsewhere in this issue).

Reducing Psychological Distress and Burden of Depression

Allostatic load, or wear and tear, imposed by a lifetime of physiologic or psychological stresses and adaptations, also seems to contribute to cognitive decline in late life, independent of the pathologic features of AD.[2,35] Chronic distress (eg, chronic or recurrent depression, hopelessness, feelings of loneliness, working long hours) in middle-aged adults and older adults is associated with increased risk of atherosclerosis, neurodegeneration, and future dementia (especially AD and VCI).[7,36–39] There is evidence that major depression may have a toxic effect on brain function.[40] Hippocampal volume deficits are larger and more strongly associated with memory deficits in people with late-onset depression than in those with early-onset depression and may suggest that these patients are more likely to develop cognitive impairment.[41] Late-onset depression may be a prodrome of late dementia and may also promote neuropathogenic processes that eventually cause dementia.[42] These findings, if replicated, have important implications for public health because of high prevalence of chronic distress and depression. Stress or distress may have a significant effect on the onset, course, and management of many, if not all, diseases.[43] Stress is associated with increased engagement in other harmful habits such as cigarette smoking and low exercise levels. Depression has been associated with increased rates of cardiovascular illness, diabetes mellitus, smoking, and hypertension.[44–46] On the other hand, personality and psychosocial factors that are associated with lower risk of dementia have also been identified. These factors include socially integrated lifestyle,

Table 2
Checklist to promote healthy brain aging: a guide for clinicians

1	Counseled regarding smoking cessation	☐
	Comments:	
2	Advised to follow guidelines proposed jointly by the American Heart Association and the American College of Sports Medicine regarding daily physical activity	☐
	Comments:	
3	Counseled regarding healthy nutrition (eg, Mediterranean diet, DASH [Dietary Approaches to Stop Hypertension] diet)	☐
	Comments:	
4	Counseled regarding the importance of intellectually challenging and creative leisure activities	☐
	Comments:	
5	Counseled regarding strategies to promote emotional resilience and reduce psychological distress and depression (eg, relaxation exercises, mindfulness-meditation practices)	☐
	Comments:	
6	Advised to maintain an active, socially integrated lifestyle	☐
	Comments:	
7	Discussed strategies to achieve and maintain optimal daily sleep	☐
	Comments:	

8	Provided education about strategies to reduce risk of serious head injury (eg, wearing seat belts, wearing helmets during contact sports, bicycling, skiing, skateboarding)	☐
	Comments:	
9	Provided education about strategies to reduce exposure to hazardous substances (eg, wearing protective clothing during the administration of pesticides, fumigants, fertilizers, and defoliants)	☐
	Comments:	
10	Provided education and counseling regarding negative health effects of alcohol consumption more than recommended as safe by the National Institute of Alcoholism and Alcohol Abuse	☐
	Comments:	
11	Provided education about importance of achieving and maintaining healthy weight to promote overall health	☐
	Comments:	
12	Discussed and implemented strategies to achieve optimal blood pressure control	☐
	Comments:	
13	Discussed and implemented strategies to achieve optimal control of dyslipidemia (eg, high cholesterol)	☐
	Comments:	
14	Discussed and implemented strategies to achieve optimal control of blood sugar/ diabetes	☐
	Comments:	
15	Discussed risks and benefits of medications, supplements, herbal remedies, and vitamins to promote brain health	☐
	Comments:	
16	Discussed and implemented secondary prevention of stroke strategies (eg, daily baby aspirin)	☐
	Comments:	

Courtesy of Center for Healthy Brain Aging, Saint Louis University School of Medicine, St Louis, MO.

conscientiousness, low neuroticism, and high extraversion (see the article by McFadden and Basting elsewhere in this issue).[47,48] Strong correlations exist between the well-being, happiness, health, and longevity of people who are emotionally and behaviorally compassionate, so long as they are not overwhelmed by helping tasks.[49] Healthy and resilient aging is more than preserving cognitive function and delaying onset of dementia. In daily life, the domains of emotional and cognitive health are inseparably linked. Thus, promoting emotional well-being and treating depression are important for overall health and more specifically for cognitive health.

STEP 5: UNDERSTANDING WHO THE TARGET POPULATION IS, WHEN TO START APPLYING THESE INTERVENTIONS, AND WHEN TO STOP

From a clinical and public health perspective, it is important to be able to predict who is at highest risk of developing future dementia and when. Although 2 risk assessment tools have been studied (1 in middle-aged adults and 1 in older adults),[50,51] more research is needed to improve these formulas and their ease of use (regarding complexity and cost) before they can be used in routine clinical practice. Using comparative genotype relative-risk information and survival data from family studies, estimates of gender-, age-, and genotype-specific risk can be generated for use in risk-assessment research that features genotype disclosure.[52] The main value of such scales and tools would be educational. Thus, a dementia risk predictor tool that is reminiscent of the coronary heart disease risk scales posted on the American Heart Association's Web site is urgently needed. VRFs (eg, obesity) in midlife may be more important than in older age because VRFs may take longer to impair neurologic function. The longer the person has VRFs, the higher that person's risk of future AD and VCI. Thus, middle-aged adults with multiple VRFs may be considered a target population for programs that promote healthy brain aging. Adults with family history of AD, especially familial AD, and adults with history of AD in both parents are also an appropriate target population for such programs. Also, understanding which individuals with MCI are at highest risk for eventually developing AD is key to the ultimate goal of delaying the onset of AD and of preventing AD.[13] Superior health at old age (85 years and older) does not guarantee protection against cognitive decline and AD. Even among the healthiest, oldest-old people (adults 85 years and older who represent the top 1%–3% of oldest-old people for health), 20% developed dementia (AD mostly) in 5 to 6 years.[53] Thus, although the effect of strategies to promote healthy brain aging in late life are unclear, prudence dictates that at least some of the strategies listed (eg, staying physically, mentally, and socially active, and optimal control of blood pressure) should be routinely recommended for adults aged 85 years and older.

Genetic Education and Counseling

Adult children of patients diagnosed with AD routinely express their own fears of developing AD in the future and often inquire about genetic testing. Approximately 0.7% to 0.9% of AD cases clearly exhibit autosomal-dominant transmission in more than 1 generation (ie, a sibling, a parent, and a grandparent also have AD).[54] Predictive genetic testing, with appropriate pre- and posttesting counseling, may be offered to at-risk individuals with an apparent autosomal-dominant inheritance of AD.[6] Adult children with family history of AD, especially children who have history of both parents having AD, may also benefit from genetic counseling.[55] Given the uncertainties surrounding the potential increased risk for AD in an individual rather than in a population, screening for APOE4 in asymptomatic individuals in the general population is not recommended.[6] For guidelines and recommendations on the application of genetics in the assessment, diagnosis, and management of patients and families with dementia, readers are referred to the article by Hsiung and Sadovnick.[54]

STEP 6: UNDERSTANDING THE POTENTIAL FOR BRAIN CHANGES (NEUROPLASTICITY), THE CAPACITY OF THE BRAIN TO GENERATE NEW BRAIN CELLS (NEUROGENESIS), AND THE CONCEPT OF COGNITIVE RESERVE

Neuroplasticity is the capacity of our brains to change with experience. Research on the biology of brain aging supports the idea that the brain is capable of changing at all ages, although this capacity declines with age. Maximizing the potential benefits of brain plasticity requires engaging adults in challenging cognitive, sensory, and motor activities on an intensive basis.[56] The rate of neurogenesis and the survival of repli-cating progenitors are strongly modified by behavioral interventions known to impinge on the rate of neurogenesis and the probability of survival of newly born neurons, including exercise, enriched experience, and learning.[57] A unique opportunity may exist in which the therapeutic stimulation of neurogenesis might contribute to func-tional repair of the adult diseased brain, before damage to whole neuronal networks has ensued. The concept of cognitive reserve (CR) describes the ability of the adult brain to sustain normal function in the face of significant disease or injury.[58] The CR capacity is probably set early in life (the first 2–3 decades) and gradually declines as the brain ages. The impact of brain diseases or injuries may be less apparent in those with a greater CR, as healthy brain tissue is able to accommodate for the lost neurons and synapses. In those with lower CR capacity, the effects of the same injury may be more readily apparent as the limited resources available in this situation become ex-pended more quickly. CR is probably determined by structural reserve (eg, larger brain size, more neurons and synapses), and functional reserve (eg, activity of specific neural circuits and synapses and the efficient use of alternative brain networks). Some risk factors (including genetic inheritance, emotional deprivation, and emotional abuse) that alter brain formation and growth may have their major effects in early life. Other risk factors related to socioeconomic status, such as smoking, malnutrition, and obesity in childhood/adulthood, may set the stage for later adulthood influences such as insulin resistance, obesity, hyperlipidemia, hypertension, diabetes, metabolic syndrome, cardiovascular, and cerebrovascular disease, all related to increased inci-dence of AD. Such findings point to the importance of taking a life-course perspective to designing interventions to delay or to prevent dementia.[59]

STEP 7: UNDERSTANDING THE DIRECTIONS THAT FUTURE RESEARCH NEEDS TO TAKE TO MAKE HEALTHY BRAIN AGING A REALITY FOR ALL

Future research may shed light on the best clinical strategies regarding the "how" and "what" of information dissemination to all adults toward reducing the incidence and prevalence of dementias and increasing healthy brain aging. The authors believe that the future lies in advances in basic research, technological developments, and progress in clinical research. Neuroscience may soon realize the promise of detecting neurodegenerative processes (eg, those involved in AD) and processes involved in cerebrovascular disease (eg, those involved in atherosclerosis), before they are behaviorally observable (eg, through change in cognition, mood, or personality), thus realizing the promise for early intervention. Discovering and targeting the path-ways mediating aging and disease susceptibility and developing therapeutic agents will allow more of the population to age with intact cognition. Some elderly persons whose brains have high densities of lesions that indicate neurodegenerative disease do not have dementia.[60] It is of utmost importance to find out how common such cases are and their relationship to healthy brain aging to help prevent treatment of presymptomatic AD in older adults who have low likelihood of developing dementia.

Dementia is not an event, but the end stage of several pathophysiologic processes. The focus needs to be shifted from the extreme category of dementia to the continuum of cognitive functioning that includes milder forms of cognitive impairment and brain at risk (eg, positive amyloid imaging scans). Also, neurodegenerative and cerebrovascular pathologies are not mutually exclusive, but interact in their contribution to cognitive impairment and dementia. Cognitive impairment is also not always the first (or main) alarm signal. These interactions need to be acknowledged when planning secondary prevention trials. The most prevalent activity throughout life is work. Future studies need to clarify whether retirement has detrimental effects on cognitive and emotional health, especially for individuals who do not have resources to maintain a high level of activity and social participation.[61] Identifying convergent mechanisms such as insulin resistance, hypoperfusion, and cerebral ischemia that may underlie co-morbid VRFs and thereby increase dementia risk will provide important insight into the causes and interdependencies of late-life dementias and may also identify novel strategies for treating and preventing these disorders.

As understanding of risk factors improves, it may be possible to personalize dementia prevention. A tool that looks simultaneously at several genetic variants, family history, lifestyle, VRFs, and vascular disease might more accurately predict who is at risk for dementia and who could benefit from more aggressive prevention efforts. Phenotypes that reflect healthy brain aging need further refinement to better understand their genetic, lifestyle, and environmental basis.[62] This refinement must be done before we can begin to understand the complex array of factors affecting healthy brain aging and brain health span. Only in the last few years has attention been paid to studying preserved cognition as an outcome in older adults. Future research needs to identify validated instruments to measure these outcomes.

Most studies to date have not included the whole spectrum of successful brain aging (cognitive, emotional, and physical health) despite the fact that the relationship between cognitive, emotional, and physical health is complex, intertwined, and may have common underlying processes. There is also an emerging realization that whenever 2 pathologies occur together, they accelerate disease. Research into the links between different proteins at the monomeric and oligomeric levels is needed to further explore these possibilities. Thus, in the future, there may be a shift away from relying on clinical categorization to make diagnoses to using sophisticated biomarkers to make diagnoses based on accumulation of various types of toxic proteins (eg, amyloid-β, τ, α-synuclein) while simultaneously detecting cerebrovascular ischemia. Future research needs to clarify whether depression contributes to the development of AD, or whether another unknown factor causes depression and AD.

STEP 8: UNDERSTANDING THE ROLE OF GOVERNMENT, HEALTH-INSURANCE COMPANIES, AND ACADEMIC INSTITUTIONS IN PROMOTING HEALTHY BRAIN AGING

The US Centers of Disease Control (CDC) in partnership with the Alzheimer's Association has proposed a set of 44 actions grounded in science and that emphasize primary prevention to achieve the long-term goal of maintaining or improving cognitive performance in all adults.[1] Each priority action is based on a detailed, scientific rationale, with implementation to be based on demonstrated effectiveness of specific interventions. This is an excellent first step but government can do more to promote healthy brain aging. For example, the evidence that long-term exposure to air pollution contributes to arterial diseases and atherosclerosis is substantial.[63] Any effort by the government to reduce air pollution thus may have health benefits besides the obvious environmental benefits. Individual VRFs (eg, hypertension, obesity, and diabetes) do not spectacularly increase the risk of AD or VCI in individual patients with any of these conditions (relative risk).[22] By contrast, as VRFs are common conditions with a high prevalence, this modest increase in risk translates into an increased attributable risk at the population level. To demonstrate a clinically significant effect of optimal control of various VRFs in a prospective RCT would be challenging in the infrastructure and financial resources required to conduct such a trial. With limited resources (financial and human), the authors think the government should avoid funding such studies and instead use the same funds to make optimal control of VRFs in primary care universal.

From an academic perspective, the practice style of most physicians is focused on medical technology and pharmaceuticals rather than prevention and wellness promotion. To change this focus requires a change in how academic institutions train physicians, and government and health-insurance companies finance preventive care involving lifestyle modification and services focused on VRF management. Academic institutions should partner the government to create a credible and user-friendly Web site on which evidence-based, state-of-the-science strategies to promote healthy brain aging are made available (and periodically updated). Peer groups and educational programs have been identified as effective ways to reach people with messages about brain health, particularly within preexisting social networks such as clubs or senior centers.[64] Health messages that build on existing perceptions, use cognitive health as a motivator for healthy behaviors, and involve community champions as advocates are viewed positively by older adults.[5]

Communities should partner academic institutions to provide regular evidence-based educational seminars on various topics to empower adults in their community to take the initiative in achieving and maintaining cognitive vitality. Such programs can also dispel the myth that old age is associated with inevitable cognitive decline and that individuals are powerless against such a future. The local community can also promote healthy brain aging by making credible resource materials/Web sites accessible to the public. A list of resources recommended by the authors is given in **Table 3**.

STEP 9: UNDERSTANDING THE ROLE OF PHYSICIANS AND INDIVIDUALS IN PROMOTING HEALTHY BRAIN AGING

Physicians, physician extenders (eg, nurse practitioners, physician assistants), and nurses can play an instrumental role in helping their patients achieve and maintain healthy brain aging. They can help by explaining that healthy lifestyle and optimal control of VRFs and vascular disease increase life expectancy and reduce the risk of cancer, heart disease, and stroke, while at the same time promoting healthy brain aging.[22,23,65–68] Health care providers (HCPs) can clarify the distinction between disease prevention and risk reduction to their patients (an important distinction in expectations for benefits). There is a gap between people realizing what is good for them (eg, never smoking, regular exercise) and making this part of their daily routine. Current recommendations generally support implementing simultaneous behavior-change interventions versus sequential or single behavior change around physical activity, diet, and so forth. Nurses can and should take a leadership role in offering evidence-based preventive care during routine office visits. HCPs can engage patients in ways that support patients' innate needs for autonomy, competence, and relatedness to improve adoption and maintenance of lifelong behavioral changes. Individuals need to understand that healthy brain cells and connections are better able

Table 3
Resources for patients that physicians can recommend to promote healthy brain aging

Types of Resources	
Books	1. Improving memory: understanding age-related memory loss. A special health report from Harvard Medical School. Boston: Harvard Health Publications; 2006. http://www.health.harvard.edu/
	2. Healthy eating. A guide to the new nutrition. A special health report from Harvard Medical School. Boston: Harvard Health Publications; 2006. http://www.health.harvard.edu/
	3. Simon HB. The no sweat exercise plan. Lose weight, get healthy, and live longer. New York: McGraw Hill; 2006
	4. Cohen GD. The mature mind: the positive power of the aging brain. New York: Basic Books; 2005
	5. Doidge N. The brain that changes itself. New York: Penguin Books; 2007
	6. Vaillant GE. Aging well. New York: Little, Brown and Company; 2002
	7. Casey A, Benson H. Mind your heart: A mind/body approach to stress management, exercise, and nutrition for heart health. New York: Free Press; 2004
Audio-CD	Weil A, Smal G. The healthy brain kit. Sounds True. Also has 52-page workbook and 35 brain-training cards
Web sites	"Maintain your brain" document is a good educational tool regarding role of lifestyle in promoting brain health and reducing risk for dementia. Available at the Alzheimer's Association Web site http://www.alz.org/national/documents/brochure_maintainyourbrain.pdf
	Tip sheets for improving memory and cognitive vitality. Available at the American Geriatric Society Foundation for Health in Aging Web site http://www.healthinaging.org/
	Information on guidelines for daily physical activity. Available at The American Heart Association Web site, which includes guidelines recommended jointly by the American Heart Association and the American College of Sports Medicine on minimum daily physical activity for adults and older adults to promote and maintain health http://www.americanheartassociation.org/
	DASH diet (Dietary Approaches to Stop Hypertension). Available at: http://www.dashdiet.org/
	Information on safe amount of alcohol consumption. National Institute of Alcohol Abuse and Alcoholism "Helping patients who drink too much". Available at: http://www.niaaa.nih.gov/
	Information on achieving and maintaining healthy weight. WIN [Weight-control Information Network]. Available at: http://www.win.niddk.nih.gov/

Courtesy of Center for Healthy Brain Aging, Saint Louis University School of Medicine, St Louis, MO.

to withstand the ravages of age, genetic vulnerabilities, environmental stresses, accidents, toxins, and disease (including AD). Small measures can turn risk factors around. Individuals need to work with their health care provider to identify resources at different levels of the environment (eg, family, community, institutions) to maximize success from interventions to promote a healthy lifestyle.

SUMMARY

To alleviate the immense burden caused by dementia, delaying onset of dementia must be a priority in clinical practice and for pragmatic research. Healthy brain aging may be related to high CR, continued intense brain activity, inherited genes, and how these genes are changed by other health conditions, lifestyle, psychosocial factors, and environmental factors. Achieving excellence in healthy brain aging requires physicians to be responsible not only to the individual patient presenting in the clinic but also to the public at large. This responsibility means a new focus on population-based outcomes in addition to individual outcomes to determine which prevention strategies are most effective and to standardize care where possible to achieve the optimal public health benefit. The simplest kinds of reforms at the clinic (eg, routine implementation of the authors' checklist in primary care) can translate into improvements at the level of population health. Advances in biomedical science that reveal underlying mechanisms of brain aging and the proliferation of new treatments to slow or reverse age-related diseases that cause cognitive decline are essential to the progress of the science of aging. Most remarkable, however, is the recurrent theme in rigorous studies that shows the importance of lifestyle modification, psychosocial factors, and control of VRFs in preserving brain function and preventing dementia. As our understanding of the myriad ways in which the forces of biology and psychosocial factors work together improves, it may not be long before healthy brain aging becomes a reality for all.

REFERENCES

1. Centers for Disease Control and Prevention and the Alzheimer's Association. The healthy brain initiative: a national public health road map to maintaining cognitive health. Chicago: Alzheimer's Association; 2007. Available at: www.cdc.gov/aging. Accessed November 29, 2009.
2. Centers for Disease Control and Prevention and the Alzheimer's Association. The healthy brain initiative: a national public health road map to maintaining cognitive health. Chicago: Alzheimer's Association; 2007. Available at: www.alz.org. Accessed November 29, 2009.
3. Hendrie HC, Albert MS, Butters MA, et al. The NIH Cognitive and Emotional Health Project: report of the Critical Evaluation Study Committee. Alzheimers Dement 2006;2:12–32.
4. Laditka SB, Corwin SJ, Laditka JN, et al. Attitudes about aging well among a diverse group of older Americans: implications for promoting cognitive health. Gerontologist 2009;49(Suppl 1):S30–9.
5. Logsdon RG, Hochhalter AK, Sharkey JR. From message to motivation: where the rubber meets the road. Gerontologist 2009;49(Suppl 1):S108–11.
6. Patterson C, Feightner JW, Garcia A, et al. Diagnosis and treatment of dementia: 1. Risk assessment and primary prevention of Alzheimer disease. CMAJ 2008; 178:548–56.
7. Middleton LE, Yaffe K. Promising strategies for the prevention of dementia. Arch Neurol 2009;66:1210–5.

8. Rabins PV. Do we know enough to begin prevention interventions for dementia? Alzheimers Dement 2007;3:S86–8.

9. Rojas-Fernandez CH, Moorhouse P. Vascular cognitive impairment. Ann Pharmacother 2009;43:1310–23.

10. Neuropathology Group of the Medical Research Council Cognitive Function and Aging Study (MRC CFAS). Pathological correlates of late-onset dementia in a multicenter, community-based population in England and Wales. Lancet 2001;357:169–75.

11. Rosenberg PB, Lyketsos C. Mild cognitive impairment: searching for the prodrome of Alzheimer's disease. World Psychiatry 2008;7:72–8.

12. Martin GM. The evolutionary substrate of aging. Arch Neurol 2002;59:1702–5.

13. Alzheimer's Association. 2009 Alzheimer's disease facts and figures. Alzheimers Dement 2009;5:234–70.

14. Perls T. Dementia-free centenarians. Exp Gerontol 2004;39:1587–93.

15. Schoenhofen EA, Wyszynski DF, Andersen S, et al. Characteristics of 32 supercentenarians. J Am Geriatr Soc 2006;54:1237–40.

16. Willcox DC, Willcox BJ, Wang N, et al. Life at the extreme limit: phenotypic characteristics of supercentenarians in Okinawa. J Gerontol A Biol Sci Med Sci 2008; 63:1201–8.

17. Brookmeyer R, Gray S, Kawas C. Projections of Alzheimer's disease in the United States and the public health impact of delaying disease onset. Am J Public Health 1998;88(9):1337–42.

18. Brookmeyer R, Johnson E, Ziegler-Graham K, et al. Forecasting the global burden of Alzheimer's disease. Alzheimers Dement 2007;3:186–91.

19. Miller M. An emerging paradigm in atherosclerosis: focus on subclinical disease. Postgrad Med 2009;121:49–59.

20. Mortimer JA, Gosche KM, Snowdon DA. Very early detection of Alzheimer neuropathology and the role of brain reserve in modifying its clinical expression. J Geriatr Psychiatry Neurol 2005;18:218–23.

21. Kivipelto M, Solomon A. Alzheimer's disease–the ways of prevention. J Nutr Health Aging 2008;12:S89–94.

22. Viswanathan A, Rocca WA, Tzourio C. Vascular risk factors and dementia. How to move forward? Neurology 2009;72:368–74.

23. Gluckman TJ, Baranowski B, Ashen D, et al. A practical and evidence-based approach to cardiovascular disease risk reduction. Arch Intern Med 2004;164: 1490–500.

24. Rogers WJ, Canto JG, Lambrew CT, et al. Temporal trends in the treatment of over 1.5 million patients with myocardial infarction in the US from 1990 through 1999: the National Registry of Myocardial infarction 1,2 and 3. J Am Coll Cardiol 2000;36:2056–63.

25. Kopunek SP, Michael KM, Shaughnessy M, et al. Cardiovascular risk in survivors of stroke. Am J Prev Med 2007;32:408–12.

26. Jencks SF, Cuerdon T, Burwen DR, et al. Quality of medical care delivered to Medicare beneficiaries: a profile at state and national levels. JAMA 2000;284: 1670–6.

27. Preis SR, Pencina MJ, Hwang SJ, et al. Trends in Cardiovascular Disease Risk Factors in individuals with and without diabetes mellitus in the Framingham Heart Study. Circulation 2009;120:212–20.

28. Reeves MJ, Rafferty AP. Healthy lifestyle characteristics among adults in the United States, 2000. Arch Intern Med 2005;165:854–7.

29. Hejl A, Hogh P, Waldemar G. Potentially reversible conditions in 1000 consecutive memory clinic patients. J Neurol Neurosurg Psychiatr 2002;73:390–4.

30. Isaac MG, Quinn R, Tabet N. Vitamin E for Alzheimer's disease and mild cognitive impairment. Cochrane Database Syst Rev 2008;(3):CD002854.

31. DeKosky ST, Williamson JD, Fitzpatrick AL, et al. Ginkgo biloba for prevention of dementia: a randomized controlled trial. JAMA 2008;300:2253–62.

32. Sesso HD, Buriing JE, Christen WG, et al. Vitamins E and C in the prevention of cardiovascular disease in men: the Physicians' Health Study II randomized controlled trial. JAMA 2008;300:2123–33.

33. Ristow M, Zarse K, Oberbach A, et al. Antioxidants prevent health-promoting effects of physical exercise in humans. Proc Natl Acad Sci U S A 2009;106:8665–70.

34. Yashodhara BM, Umakanth S, Pappachan JM, et al. Omega-3 fatty acids: a comprehensive review of their role in health and disease. Postgrad Med J 2009;85:84–90.

35. Wilson RS, Arnold SE, Schneider JA, et al. Chronic distress, age-related neuropathology, and late-life dementia. Psychosom Med 2007;69:47–53.

36. Whipple MO, Lewis TT, Sutton-Tyrrell K, et al. Hopelessness, depressive symptoms, and carotid atherosclerosis in women: the Study of Women's Health Across the Nation (SWAN) heart study. Stroke 2009;40:3166–72.

37. Tsolaki M, Kounti F, Karamavrou S. Severe psychological stress in elderly individuals: a proposed model of neurodegeneration and its implications. Am J Alzheimers Dis Other Demen 2009;24:85–94.

38. Tilvis RS, Kahonen-Vare MH, Jolkkonen J, et al. Predictors of cognitive decline and mortality of aged people over a 10-year period. J Gerontol A Biol Sci Med Sci 2004;59:M268–74.

39. Virtanen M, Singh-Manoux A, Ferrie JE, et al. Long working hours and cognitive function: the Whitehall II study. Am J Epidemiol 2009;169:596–605.

40. Gorwood P, Corruble E, Falissard B, et al. Toxic effects of depression on brain function: impairment of delayed recall and the cumulative length of depressive disorder in a large sample of depressed outpatients. Am J Psychiatry 2008;165:731–9.

41. Ballmaier M, Narr KL, Toga AW, et al. Hippocampal morphology and distinguishing late-onset from early-onset elderly depression. Am J Psychiatry 2008;165:229–37.

42. Tsuno N, Homma A. What is the association between depression and Alzheimer's disease. Expert Rev Neurother 2009;9:1667–76.

43. Selhub EV. Stress and distress in clinical practice: a mind-body approach. Nutr Clin Care 2002;5:182–90.

44. Carney RM, Blumenthal JA, Stein PK, et al. Depression, heart rate variability and acute myocardial infarction. Circulation 2001;104:2024–8.

45. Lustman PJ, Griffith LS, Gavard JA, et al. Depression in adults with diabetes. Diabetes Care 1992;15:1631–9.

46. Rutledge T, Hogan BE. A quantitative review of prospective evidence linking psychological factors with hypertension development. Psychosom Med 2002;64:758–66.

47. Wilson RS, Schneider JA, Arnold SE, et al. Conscientiousness and the incidence of Alzheimer disease and mild cognitive impairment. Arch Gen Psychiatry 2007;64:1204–12.

48. Wang HX, Karp A, Herlitz A, et al. Personality and lifestyle in relation to dementia incidence. Neurology 2009;72:253–9.

49. Post SG. Altruism, happiness, and health: It's good to be good. Int J Behav Med 2005;12(2):66–77.
50. Kivipelto M, Ngandu T, Laatikainen T, et al. Risk score for the prediction of dementia risk in 20 years among middle aged people: a longitudinal, population-based study. Lancet Neurol 2006;5:735–41.
51. Barnes DE, Covinsky KE, Whitmer RA, et al. Predicting risk of dementia in older adults: the late-life dementia risk index. Neurology 2009;73:173–9.
52. Cupples LA, Farrer LA, Sadovnick AD, et al. Estimating risk curves for first-degree relatives of patients with Alzheimer's disease: the REVEAL study. Genet Med 2004;6:192–6.
53. McNeal MG, Zapeparsi S, Camicioli R, et al. Predictors of healthy brain aging. J Gerontol A Biol Sci Med Sci 2001;56:B294–301.
54. Hsiung GYR, Sadovnick AD. Genetics and dementia: risk factors, diagnosis and management. Alzheimers Dement 2007;3:418–27.
55. Jayadev S, Steinbart EJ, Chi YY, et al. Conjugal Alzheimer disease: risk in children when both parents have Alzheimer disease. Arch Neurol 2008;65:373–8.
56. Mahncke HW, Bronstone A, Merzenich MM. Brain plasticity and functional losses in the aged: scientific bases for a novel intervention. Prog Brain Res 2006;157:81–109.
57. Galvan V, Bredesen DE. Neurogenesis in the adult brain: implications for Alzheimer's disease. CNS Neurol Disord Drug Targets 2007;6:303–10.
58. Stern Y. Cognitive reserve. Neuropsychologia 2009;47:2015–28.
59. Gatz M, Prescott CA, Pedersen NL. Lifestyle risk and delaying factors. Alzheimer Dis Assoc Disord 2006;20(3 Suppl 2):S84–8.
60. Savva GM, Wharton SB, Ince PG, et al. Age, neuropathology, and dementia. N Engl J Med 2009;360:2302–9.
61. Lyketsos C. Commentary on "The NIH Cognitive and Emotional Health Project Report of the Critical Evaluation Study Committee." What would be the effect of raising the retirement age by five years on the cognitive and emotional health of individuals age 65 and older? Alzheimers Dement 2006;2:86–8.
62. Willcox BJ, Willcox DC, Ferrucci L. Secrets of healthy aging and longevity from exceptional survivors around the globe: lessons from octogenarians to supercentenarians. J Gerontol A Biol Sci Med Sci 2008;63:1181–5.
63. Brook RD, Franklin B, Cascio W, et al. Air pollution and cardiovascular disease: a statement for healthcare professionals from the Expert Panel on Population and Prevention Science of the American Heart Association. Circulation 2004;109:2655–71.
64. Friedman DB, Laditka JN, Hunter R, et al. Getting the message out about brain health: a cross-cultural comparison of older adults' media awareness and communication needs on how to maintain a healthy brain. Gerontologist 2009;49(Suppl 1):S50–60.
65. World Cancer Research Fund/American Institute for Cancer Research. The second expert report. food, nutrition, physical activity, and the prevention of cancer: a global perspective. Washington, DC: AICR; 2009.
66. Dimsdale JE. Psychological stress and cardiovascular disease. J Am Coll Cardiol 2008;51(13):1237–46.
67. Vieweg WVR, Pandurangi AK. The relation of stress and psychiatric illnesses to coronary heart disease. Acta Psychiatr Scand 2006;113:241–4.
68. Fraser GE, Shavlik DJ. Ten years of life: is it a matter of choice? Arch Intern Med 2001;161:1645–52.

Cardiovascular Risk Factors, Cerebrovascular Disease Burden, and Healthy Brain Aging

Leon Flicker, MB BS, PhD, FRACP[a,b,*]

KEYWORDS

- Healthy brain aging • Cardiovascular risk factors
- Cognitive impairment • Depression

Healthy brain functioning can be defined as the absence of chronic mental diseases, high cognitive functioning, and unimpaired ability to actively engage with life. However, it has become clear that these 3 facets are not tightly interwoven and that older people can still be actively engaged with social activities even in the presence of major cognitive impairment.[1] Nevertheless, healthy brain aging implies the absence of major mental illness, particularly of those conditions that often accompany the aging process: depression and cognitive impairment. This article reviews the evidence that cardiovascular risk factors increase the risk of cognitive impairment and depression, potential mechanisms by which cerebrovascular burden influences cognitive health, how this might change clinical practice and public health policy, and key gaps in our current knowledge (**Table 1**).

CARDIOVASCULAR RISK FACTORS AND COGNITIVE IMPAIRMENT

Serious cognitive impairment, involving memory and other cognitive abilities, that interferes with an older person's social or occupational activities, fulfils criteria for dementia. It is now also realized that cognitive impairment, not fulfilling criteria for dementia (CIND), may be more common than dementia. In 1 community-based study the prevalence of CIND was found to be 16.8%, whereas the prevalence of all types of

---

[a] Department of Geriatric Medicine, School of Medicine and Pharmacology, University of Western Australia, Perth, Australia
[b] Western Australian Centre for Health and Ageing, CMR, Western Australian Institute for Medical Research, Perth, Australia
* Department of Geriatric Medicine, Royal Perth Hospital, Box X2213 GPO, Perth, WA 6001, Australia.
E-mail address: leon.flicker@uwa.edu.au

Clin Geriatr Med 26 (2010) 17–27
doi:10.1016/j.cger.2009.12.005
0749-0690/10/$ – see front matter © 2010 Elsevier Inc. All rights reserved.

Table 1 Cardiovascular risk factors and potential mechanisms by which they may affect the brain	
Cardiovascular Risk Factor	**Potential Mechanisms**
Advancing age	Large vessel cerebral infarcts
Family history	Small vessel cerebral infarcts
Hypertension	Cerebral hemorrhage
Diabetes mellitus	Cerebral microhemorrhages
Hyperlipidemia	Chronic cerebral hypoperfusion
Smoking	Secondary neuronal degeneration
Obesity	Neuronal dysfunction with neurotramsmitter changes
Hyperhomocysteinemia	Endothelial dysfunction
Atrial fibrillation	Inflammatory mediated changes
Sedentary lifestyle	Oxidative stress
	Advanced glycation end products
	Increased production or decreased clearance of β-amyloid protein in the brain

dementia combined was 8%.[2] The conditions identified within this category of CIND in this study included delirium, alcohol use, drug intoxication, depression, psychiatric disorders, memory impairment associated with the aging process and intellectual disability. More recently this category of cognitive impairment not fulfilling criteria for dementia has undergone reclassification with many people within this category labeled as mild cognitive impairment (MCI),[3] with subtypes of amnestic and nonamnestic MCI. However, effective treatment strategies for MCI have not been developed.

The types of dementia manifest in older people include dementia in Alzheimer disease (AD) (either early or late onset), vascular dementia (VD), and dementia in other diseases, as categorized by the World Health Organization ICD 10.[4] More recently dementia with Lewy bodies is commonly diagnosed.[5] However, recent neuropathologic studies of older people who have died with dementia, have revealed that pure forms of these disease entities are relatively uncommon, and many older people manifest multiple neuropathologies that lead to cognitive dysfunction.[6] For people with dementia who are older than 80 years, neuropathologic abnormalities are not as clear cut, and many older people who die with dementia, do not have severe Alzheimer or vascular pathology.[7] Because of these pathologic uncertainties, it is still reasonable to discuss risk factors that are associated with worsening cognitive impairment or dementia and not specific types of dementia.

Complicating this picture further is our dearth of knowledge in some key areas. Risk factors for types of dementia, other than AD and VD, have not been identified. The risk factors for VD have largely been extrapolated from the risk factors for stroke, and these risk factors have been more clearly elucidated. Risk factors for stroke can be classified as traditional or novel, and modifiable or nonmodifiable. The nonmodifiable risk factors include age, sex, ethnicity, and family history. Modifiable traditional risk factors include hypertension, diabetes, hyperlipidemia, atrial fibrillation, smoking, obesity, and carotid artery disease. Novel risk factors include hyperhomocysteinemia, hypercoagulable states, and selective biomarkers.[8]

In the last 15 years some of these traditional cardiovascular risk factors have not only been found to predict VD but also AD. It is now accepted that hypertension is a risk factor for AD. Initial observational studies, for example, Skoog and colleagues,[9] showed that hypertension some 15 years before the onset of dementia not only predicted an increased risk of VD but also AD. Unexpectedly, the group of subjects with AD did not seem to have a greater prevalence of hypertension after the onset of the disease. Subsequently, not only was midlife hypertension confirmed as a risk factor for AD but also hypercholesterolemia[10] and diabetes mellitus.[11] Smoking was initially believed to be protective for the development of AD, based on case-control studies. These data were found to be misleading and prone to survivorship bias compared with cohort studies that show a positive association between smoking and AD[12]; this association has been confirmed by a comprehensive meta-analysis.[13] Further evidence for a biologic basis for this association includes the demonstration of abnormalities in the gray matter of the brain of smokers almost identical to that found in people with early AD.[14] A recent observational study of people with AD, identified by population-based sampling, showed that the presence of atrial fibrillation, systolic hypertension, and angina were associated with more rapid cognitive and functional decline.[15]

The evidence is now convincing that midlife vascular risk factors are associated with AD, VD, and the more general entity of cognitive impairment in later life. Unfortunately this evidence is entirely based on observational studies, and there is relatively little trial evidence that interventions based on ameliorating these cardiovascular risk factors will reduce the risk of dementia or cognitive impairment. The use of antihypertensives has been the most studied, but a recent meta-analysis[16] failed to find conclusive evidence of a reduction in the rates of dementia with treatment. This meta-analysis concluded that the included studies were biased because of the large number of control subjects who required treatment with antihypertensives,[16] which may have diluted any treatment effect. However, the inclusion of 1 additional randomized trial in another meta-analysis (which included patients with previous cerebrovascular disease) showed a 13% reduction in the rate of incident dementia.[17] Other treatments that have been reported to reduce the incidence of stroke have not been shown to reduce the rates of either VD or vascular cognitive impairment. These treatments include anticoagulation for those patients in atrial fibrillation, antiplatelet agents, and treatment of diabetes mellitus and hyperlipidemia.[18]

Other common noncerebral manifestations of cardiovascular risk factors may also be associated with cognitive impairment. For example, cardiac failure, usually a product of ischemic heart disease, may be associated with deficits in attention and memory[19] and structural abnormalities on brain imaging.[20] Coronary artery disease has been demonstrated in 1 study to be associated with nonamnestic MCI.[21] It is unclear whether the association between cardiac disease and cognitive dysfunctioning is a result of the probable frequent coexisting cerebrovascular disease or is a product of chronic low cardiac output (or both).

CARDIOVASCULAR RISK FACTORS AND DEPRESSION

A recent review has summarized our current understanding of the complex interrelationships between cardiovascular risk factors and depression.[22] The evidence for such relationships is reinforced by the observation that one-third of stroke survivors will experience depressive symptoms. The onset of depression has been associated with other vascular risk factors such as diabetes mellitus. Depression has been correlated with an increased number of white matter lesions, which represents cumulative vascular damage to the brain. It is also known that depression occurs in about one-third of patients who survive myocardial infarction.[23] Closely related to this association, depression has also been shown to be an independent risk factor for cardiovascular and cerebrovascular events.

In a study of 5439 men older than 70 years of age,[24] cross-sectional relationships were observed between depression and diabetes mellitus, heart disease, stroke, and smoking. However, the most powerful effects seemed to be high plasma homocysteine and triglycerides. In another study, based on the same cohort,[25] 1 of the methylenetetrahydrofolate reductase (MTHFR) genotypes (C677T), was found to be associated with increased levels of homocysteine, and increased levels of homocysteine were in turn associated with depression. Based on the concept of Mendelian randomization, which allows causal inferences to be made on observational data, homocysteine was considered to very likely be implicated in the development of depression. It was concluded that lowering homocysteine levels by 1.4 μmol/L could potentially reduce the risk of depression by about 20% in the overall population, independent of individual genotypes. Unfortunately trial evidence is not yet available to confirm this hypothesis.

In a case-control study of adults more than 50 years of age,[26] a cerebrovascular risk factor score, based on the sum of severities of hypertension, coronary artery disease, diabetes mellitus, atrial fibrillation, left-ventricular hypertrophy, and smoking, was found to be strongly associated with the risk of suicide even after adjustment for age, sex, physical illness burden, functional impairment, and the presence of depressive disorder. Possible explanations for these finding are greater intensity of depressive symptoms in subjects with cerebrovascular risk factors, or changes in central monoaminergic functioning, or loss of the brain's frontal circuits leading to a greater likelihood of impulsive acts.

What trial evidence is available that treatment of vascular risk factor decreases the risk of depression? Relatively little evidence has been accumulated to test this hypothesis partly because it is difficult to withhold treatment of cardiovascular risk factors for a myriad of other benefits. The lack of this evidence, and indirect ecological evidence demonstrating no correlation between the prevalence of vascular risk factors and depression with age, has caused some commentators to question whether vascular risk factors are actually part of the causal pathway.[27] More often the hypothesis that depression itself may be another cardiovascular risk factors has been evaluated. For example, in patients with diabetes who were managed by medical practices that had been randomized to have enhanced depression management algorithms, subsequent all-cause mortality was reduced.[28] This implies that depression is a significant factor in itself in the progression of vascular disease.

POTENTIAL MECHANISMS BY WHICH CEREBROVASCULAR BURDEN INFLUENCES THE HEALTHY BRAIN

The entity of vascular cognitive impairment has been proposed to encompass the many and varied mechanisms by which vascular risk factors lead to cognitive dysfunction.[29] The traditional concept of VD, reflected in the earlier term multi-infarct dementia, has been expanded to include a wide range of syndromes including subcortical ischemic vascular dementia (Binswanger disease), strategic-infarct dementia, hypoperfusion dementia, hemorrhagic dementia, and dementias resulting from specific arteriopathies. Furthermore, there is recognition that there may be a vascular element in the etiology of degenerative dementias such as AD. It is now realized that vascular cognitive impairment without dementia is the most prevalent subgroup of vascular cognitive impairment in those less than 85 years of age.[30]

The association between cardiovascular risk factors and AD has raised several competing hypotheses. A dominant view is that vascular factors potentiate worsening of brain pathology after other mechanisms have led to the initial deposition of abnormal material, including plaques and tangles, the hallmarks of AD. The alternate hypothesis is that vascular abnormalities may be the primary event. There is some evidence for the latter hypothesis in that subjects who have AD, but no other apparent vascular risk factors, have alteration in the dynamics of vascular supply. For example flow-mediated dilatation of the brachial artery was reduced compared with controls and correlated with the degree of severity of AD.[31] Another study showed that in patients with AD or MCI, discernible changes were detected in endothelial function, compared with controls of similar age.[32] Both these studies imply that vascular and endothelial dysfunction may be the primary event, before the onset of the clinical syndrome of AD.

The presence of coronary artery disease, which in turn is associated with cardiovascular risk factors, is also associated with brain abnormalities. There is now evidence that, in patients with coronary artery disease, there was loss of gray matter volume in multiple parts of the brain, including some that play a major role in cognitive function and behavior.[33] This was an unexpected finding as direct ischemic damage would have been thought to have been due to involvement of the small penetrating arteries of the brain and therefore produce white matter abnormalities as opposed to gray matter destruction. Gray matter losses were detected in the left medial frontal lobe (including the cingulate), precentral and postcentral cortex, right temporal lobe and left middle temporal gyrus, and left precuneus and posterior cingulate in those subjects with coronary artery disease. These findings help explain the observations that patients with coronary artery disease show cognitive and behavioral changes consistent with disruption of the anterior and posterior association cortex. Lesions to the medial portions of the frontal cortex have been associated with apathy and decreased initiative. These regions are also part of networks involved in processes relevant to working memory, attentional resource allocation, reaction time, and episodic information. Potential pathophysiologic mechanisms for these changes are not clear, but might result from an enhanced effect on neurodegeneration, primary ischemic damage on the gray matter, secondary gray matter changes as a result of white matter disease, or other as yet unidentified factors.

Studies investigating gray matter changes in patients with congestive heart failure (CHF) have observed a more extensive pattern of gray matter loss: right and left insular cortex, putamen and globus pallidus, parahippocampal and fusiform gyri, thalamus, cingulate cortex, cerebellar cortex, ventral frontal, deep anterior parietal, superior lateral frontal, posterior parietal/occipital cortex, and superior temporal cortex.[34] Marked functional abnormalities in the left mid/posterior cingulate have also been reported among patients with CHF.[35] In another case-control study[20] patients with CHF (left-ventricular ejection fraction <40%) and controls without CHF, all free of clinically significant cognitive impairment, were assessed using a cognitive battery, a depression scale and semi-quantitative magnetic resonance imaging. The CHF patients had lower scores on the cognitive battery with significantly lower scores on visuospatial, executive function, visual memory, and verbal learning tasks. Right medial temporal lobe atrophy was more prominent in patients with CHF and left medial temporal lobe atrophy and deep white matter hyperintensities showed moderate association with cognitive scores in patients with CHF.

Individual vascular risk factors may be associated with specific pathologic abnormalities. For example, smokers, when compared with age-matched controls, have been demonstrated to have decreased gray matter density in the posterior cingulate and precuneus, right thalamus, and frontal cortex compared with nonsmokers.[14] These regions have also been involved in patients suffering from incipient AD.

Another specific risk factor for dementia for which potential etiologic mechanisms have recently been elucidated is the presence of diabetes mellitus. A recent twin study has found that diabetes mellitus is a risk factor for AD and VD.[36] Using a co-twin analysis the investigators were able to adjust for the effects of genetic and shared familial environmental factors. This adjustment attenuated the effect of late-life diabetes mellitus but there was more than a doubling of the risk of dementia associated with the presences of midlife diabetes mellitus (odds ratio [OR] 2.41, 95% confidence interval [CI] 1.05–5.51), suggesting a specific effect at the time of midlife. The effect of diabetes mellitus on the risk of AD seems to be additive to the effects of the presence of a apolipoprotein E ε4 allele,[37] which is also known to be a risk factor for AD. In those patients with type 2 diabetes mellitus, hospitalization for hypoglycemic episodes was associated with an increased risk of dementia and this risk increased with the number of episodes,[38] raising the possibility that hyperinsulinemia may be involved in the pathogenesis of AD. Other potential mechanisms that have been implicated with the presence of diabetes mellitus include microvascular infarcts and inflammation (as evidenced by increased cortical interleukin 6 on autopsy specimens).[39] Another study has also observed specific abnormalities of hippocampal function associated with the presence of diabetes mellitus compared with direct ischemia.[40]

The mechanisms by which vascular factors may increase the risk of depression is also obscure. There has been considerable interest in this area following the seminal work by Alexopoulos and colleagues[41] who argued "that cerebrovascular disease can predispose, precipitate, or perpetuate a depressive syndrome in many elderly patients…" This has led to the concept of vascular depression, with possible factors mediating this nexus including autonomic dysfunction, platelet activation, activation of the hypothalamic pituitary axis, endothelial dysfunction, and inflammatory factors such as cytokines. Whether this is secondary to loss of neuronal tissue or cellular dysfunctioning with resultant neurotransmitter abnormalities is uncertain. There may also be a role for shared genetic and environmental factors, such as smoking and diet (especially involving homocysteine metabolism). Depression in later life has been associated with a relative loss of frontal lobe tissue and symmetry,[42] possibly secondary to concomitant subcortical vascular disease. However, this association has not been detected in all studies.[43]

CHANGING CLINICAL PRACTICE AND PUBLIC HEALTH POLICY

The focus of this article is on "medical" measures as lifestyle interventions such as increased physical activity and dietary interventions are dealt with elsewhere in this edition of *Geriatric Clinics*. However, it is widely accepted that diet and physical activity are potent interventions to alter the risk pattern for many older adults. Although incomplete, there is now observational evidence that vascular risk factors are associated with an unhealthy brain manifested by cognitive impairment and depression. Furthermore, the amelioration and treatment of cardiovascular risk factors have considerable other benefits, including decreased mortality and morbidity form cardiac disease and stroke. It is very likely that the treatment of cardiovascular risk factors will have additional benefits on the brain, decreasing the risk of cognitive impairment and depression although there is as yet not sufficient randomized trial evidence to support this, in contrast to the considerable evidence that exists for stroke, for example. Despite this, smoking cessation is clearly important, as the observational evidence linking smoking to numerous deleterious outcomes, including cognition and depression is very strong.

Treatment of hypertension in middle-aged and older adults is uncontroversial with numerous studies looking at the use of antihypertensives as an intervention. For example, in a recent Cochrane review[44] that summarized 15 trials (24,055 subjects older than 60 years) with moderate to severe hypertension, treatment reduced total mortality (relative risk [RR] 0.90 [0.84, 0.97]) and cardiovascular morbidity and mortality (RR 0.72 [0.68, 0.77]). In the 3 trials restricted to persons with isolated systolic hypertension the benefit was similar. In very elderly patients ($\geq$ 80 years) the reduction in total cardiovascular mortality and morbidity was similar (RR 0.75 [0.65, 0.87]) but there was no reduction in total mortality (RR 1.01 [0.90, 1.13]). The HYVET study,[45] which specifically examined patients older than 80 years, reported its results after it was terminated early because of a clear benefit of the active treatment arm. The group treated with the diuretic indapamide, plus if necessary the angiotensin-converting-enzyme inhibitor perindopril, showed more significant improvements than the placebo group. After 2 years of treatment there was a 30% reduction in the rate of stroke (95% CI −1 to 51), a 39% reduction in deaths from stroke (95% CI 1–62), a 21% reduction in death from any cause (95% CI 4–35) and a 64% reduction in the rate of heart failure (95% CI 42–78). The excellent results of treatment in these highly monitored controlled trials may not be able to be replicated in routine clinical practice in patients with frailty, multiple comorbidities, and functional impairments.

A recent systematic review has failed to find convincing evidence for antihypertensives on the incidence of dementia[16] in those subjects without prior cerebrovascular disease. This systematic review synthesized the results of 4 trials, including 15,936 hypertensive subjects. The average age was 75.4 years. The combined result of the 4 trials reporting incidence of dementia indicated no significant difference between treatment and placebo OR of 0.89 (95% CI 0.74–1.07) but there was considerable heterogeneity between the trials. The combined results from the 3 trials reporting change in the Mini Mental State Examination (MMSE) may have indicated a benefit from treatment (weighted mean difference 0.42, 95% CI 0.30–0.53). Whether the effect of antihypertensives in decreasing the risk of cognitive decline is most apparent in a subgroup of older people, for example, those who have already sustained cerebrovascular damage, or with the use of specific antihypertensives, is unclear. The significant heterogeneity between studies suggests that further studies are required to determine which class of antihypertensive is most effective and who benefits most. It is very likely that studies with dementia incidence as an outcome will need to be very large to detect an effect of 10%. However, the cognitive benefits may be shared by greater numbers of older people, not just those who progress to dementia, which has been suggested by the current trial evidence.

The treatment of hypercholesterolemia is uncontroversial for those individuals who have vascular disease. The best studied medications are the so-called statin class of drugs. It seems that they are likely to reduce mortality and the occurrence of major coronary and cerebrovascular events in patients with cardiovascular risk factors, with or without overt cardiac disease.[46] There is evidence that they reduce stroke recurrence.[47] However, it seems that statins do not specifically alter the risk of development of dementia. In a recent Cochrane review,[48] 2 trials were identified with 26,340 participants. There was no difference in incidence of dementia or performance on cognitive testing between the active and placebo groups. This represents considerable evidence of no effect. Besides the cardiovascular benefits of the statin medications, there are probably also cardiovascular benefits for dietary advice to lower dietary fat intake.[49]

Diabetes mellitus is a known risk factor for vascular diseases and is increasingly being recognized as a risk factor for cognitive impairment and depression. The UK

Prospective Diabetes Study[50] found benefits from intensive treatment of type 2 diabetes mellitus. The risk of any diabetes-related end point, including death, myocardial infarction, stroke or amputation, blindness or cataract, was reduced by 12% with more intensive treatment. However, at this stage there is no convincing evidence that intensive treatment of diabetes mellitus reduces the risk of cognitive impairment[51] or depression. However, there may be benefits of more intensive treatment of depression in people with diabetes mellitus. In patients with diabetes, who were managed by medical practices that had been randomized to have enhanced depression management algorithms, subsequent all-cause mortality was reduced.[28]

One of the major public health issues in this complex subject is not that the evidence of benefits is lacking but the penetration of known effective treatments to older people most at risk is poor. The health benefits, not just the effects on the brain, have been identified for many years. There is surprisingly poor uptake and adherence to simple measures such as antihypertensive therapy.[52] As in many areas in the treatment of older people, therapeutic nihilism, on the part of the doctor and the patient, may deprive the patient of healthy brain benefits.

KEY GAPS IN RESEARCH

There is strong observational evidence that mid- and late-life cardiovascular risk factors increase the risk of development of unhealthy brain, and in particular cognitive impairment and depression. Currently there is a lack of evidence that more aggressive treatments of these risk factors results in a healthier brain. Because of the large number of benefits associated with treatment of cardiovascular risk factors, such trials are becoming increasingly difficult to perform with a large number of the control subjects receiving unblinded interventions because of worsening clinical state. This contamination between the randomized groups makes the performance of trials difficult. It is becoming increasingly unlikely that specific trials of interventions for cardiovascular risk factors for brain outcomes will be performed. Every new trial of risk factor interventions should include cognitive and mood outcome measures. This is an easy measure to institute and would allow these effects to be determined as secondary outcomes for these studies and provide an evidence base for what is becoming an emerging consensus of benefits to the brain from amelioration of cardiovascular risk factors. Perhaps even more important are trials of increasing detection and management of cardiovascular risk factors in older people and subsequent adherence to medications.

SUMMARY

Cardiovascular risk factors have been associated with an increased risk for the development of an unhealthy brain in later life. Observational studies support a link between cardiovascular risk factors and cognitive impairment and depression. Level A evidence evaluating interventions for cardiovascular risk factors for the outcomes of cognition and depression have either been negative or inconclusive. Nevertheless, as these measures have many other health benefits, it is currently prudent to recommend targeting these risk factors at least partly to decrease the risk of developing an unhealthy brain.

REFERENCES

1. Flicker L, Lautenschlager NT, Almeida OP. Healthy mental ageing. J Br Menopause Soc 2006;12:92–6.

2. Graham JE, Rockwood K, Beattie BL, et al. Prevalence and severity of cognitive impairment with and without dementia in an elderly population. Lancet 1997;349: 1793–6.

3. Petersen RC, Doody R, Kurz A, et al. Current concepts in mild cognitive impairment. Arch Neurol 2001;58:1985–92.

4. World Health Organization. The ICD-10 classification of mental and behavioural disorders: clinical descriptions and diagnostic guidelines. Geneva, Switzerland: World Health Organization; 1992. p. 42–56.

5. McKeith IG, Dickson DW, Lowe J, et al. Diagnosis and management of dementia with Lewy bodies: third report of the DLB consortium. Neurology 2005;65: 1863–72.

6. Jellinger KA. Morphologic diagnosis of "vascular dementia" – a critical update. J Neurol Sci 2008;270:1–12.

7. Savva GM, Wharton SB, Ince PG, et al. Medical research council cognitive function and ageing study. Age, neuropathology, and dementia. N Engl J Med 2009; 360:2302–9.

8. Romero JR, Morris J, Pikula A. Stroke prevention: modifying risk factors. Ther Adv Cardiovasc Dis 2008;2:287–303.

9. Skoog I, Lernfelt B, Landahl S, et al. 15-year longitudinal study of blood pressure and dementia. Lancet 1996;347:1141–5.

10. Kivipelto M, Helkala EL, Laakso MP, et al. Midlife vascular risk factors and Alzheimer's disease in later life: longitudinal, population based study. BMJ 2001; 322(7300):1447–51.

11. Luchsinger JA, Tang MX, Stern Y, et al. Diabetes mellitus and risk of Alzheimer's disease and dementia with stroke in a multiethnic cohort. Am J Epidemiol 2001; 154:635–41.

12. Almeida OP, Hulse GK, Lawrence D, et al. Smoking as a risk factor for Alzheimer's disease: contrasting evidence from a systematic review of case–control and cohort studies. Addiction 2002;97:15–28.

13. Anstey KJ, von Sanden C, Salim A, et al. Smoking as a risk factor for dementia and cognitive decline: a meta-analysis of prospective studies. Am J Epidemiol 2007;66:367–78.

14. Almeida OP, Garrido GJ, Lautenschlager NT, et al. Smoking is associated with reduced cortical regional gray matter density in brain regions associated with incipient Alzheimer disease. Am J Geriatr Psychiatry 2008;16:92–8.

15. Mielke MM, Rosenberg PB, Tschanz J, et al. Vascular factors predict rate of progression in Alzheimer disease. Neurology 2007;69:1850–8.

16. McGuinness B, Todd S, Passmore P, et al. Blood pressure lowering in patients without prior cerebrovascular disease for prevention of cognitive impairment and dementia. Cochrane Database Syst Rev 2009;(4):CD004034.

17. Peters R, Beckett N, Forette F, et al. Incident dementia and blood pressure lowering in the Hypertension in the Very Elderly Trial Cognitive Function Assessment (HYVET-COG): a double-blind, placebo controlled trial. Lancet Neurol 2008; 7:683–9.

18. Birks J, Flicker L. Investigational treatments for vascular cognitive impairment. Expert Opin Investig Drugs 2007;16:647–58.

19. Almeida OP, Flicker L. The mind of a failing heart: a systematic review of the association between congestive heart failure and cognitive functioning. Intern Med J 2001;31:290–5.

20. Beer C, Ebenezer E, Fenner S, et al. Contributors to cognitive impairment in congestive heart failure: a pilot case-control study. Intern Med J 2009;39:600–5.

21. Roberts RO, Knopman DS, Geda YE, et al. Coronary heart disease is associated with non-amnestic mild cognitive impairment. Neurobiol Aging 2008. [Epub ahead of print].

22. Teper E, O'Brien JT. Vascular factors and depression. Int J Geriatr Psychiatry 2008;23:993–1000.

23. Thombs BD, Bass EB, Ford DE, et al. Prevalence of depression in survivors of acute myocardial infarction. J Gen Intern Med 2006;21:30–8.

24. Almeida OP, Flicker L, Norman P, et al. Association of cardiovascular risk factors and disease with depression in later life. Am J Geriatr Psychiatry 2007;15:506–13.

25. Almeida OP, McCaul K, Hankey GJ, et al. Homocysteine and depression in later life. Arch Gen Psychiatry 2008;65:1286–94.

26. Chan SS, Lyness JM, Conwell Y. Do cerebrovascular risk factors confer risk for suicide in later life? A case-control study. Am J Geriatr Psychiatry 2007;15:541–4.

27. Almeida OP. Vascular depression: myth or reality? Int Psychogeriatr 2008;20: 645–52.

28. Bogner HR, Morales KH, Post EP, et al. Diabetes, depression, and death: a randomized controlled trial of a depression treatment program for older adults based in primary care (PROSPECT). Diabetes Care 2007;30:3005–10.

29. O'Brien JT, Erkinjuntti T, Reisberg B, et al. Vascular cognitive impairment. Lancet Neurol 2003;2:89–98.

30. Rockwood K, Wentzel C, Hachinski V, et al. Prevalence and outcomes of vascular cognitive impairment. Neurology 2000;54:447–51.

31. Dede DS, Yavuz B, Yavuz BB, et al. Assessment of endothelial function in Alzheimer's disease: is Alzheimer's disease a vascular disease? J Am Geriatr Soc 2007;55:1613–7.

32. Khalil Z, LoGiudice D, Khodr B, et al. Impaired peripheral endothelial microvascular responsiveness in Alzheimer's disease. J Alzheimers Dis 2007;11:25–32.

33. Almeida OP, Garrido GJ, Beer C, et al. Coronary heart disease is associated with regional grey matter volume loss: implications for cognitive function and behaviour. Intern Med J 2008;38:599–606.

34. Woo MA, Macey PM, Fonarow GC, et al. Regional brain gray matter loss in heart failure. J Appl Phys 2003;95:677–84.

35. Woo MA, Macey PM, Keens PT, et al. Functional abnormalities in brain areas that mediate autonomic nervous system control in advanced heart failure. J Card Fail 2005;11:437–46.

36. Xu W, Qiu C, Gatz M, et al. Mid- and late-life diabetes in relation to the risk of dementia: a population-based twin study. Diabetes 2009;58:71–7.

37. Irie F, Fitzpatrick AL, Lopez OL, et al. Enhanced risk of Alzheimer disease in persons with type 2 diabetes and APOE ε4: the cardiovascular health study cognition study. Arch Neurol 2008;65:89–93.

38. Whitmer RA, Karter AJ, Yaffe K, et al. Hypoglycemic episodes and risk of dementia in older patients with type 2 diabetes mellitus. JAMA 2009;301: 1565–72.

39. Sonnen JA, Larson EB, Brickell K, et al. Different patterns of cerebral injury in dementia with or without diabetes. Arch Neurol 2009;66:315–22.

40. Wu W, Brickman AM, Luchsinger J, et al. The brain in the age of old: the hippocampal formation is targeted differentially by diseases of late life. Ann Neurol 2008;64:698–706.

41. Alexopoulos GS, Meyers BS, Young RC, et al. "Vascular depression" hypothesis. Arch Gen Psychiatry 1997;54:915–22.

42. Almeida OP, Burton EJ, Ferrier N, et al. Depression with late onset is associated with right frontal lobe atrophy. Psychol Med 2003;33:675–81.

43. Rainer MK, Mucke HA, Zehetmayer S, et al. Data from the VITA Study do not support the concept of vascular depression. Am J Geriatr Psychiatry 2006;14: 531–7.

44. Musini VM, Tejani AM, Bassett K, et al. Pharmacotherapy for hypertension in the elderly. Cochrane Database Syst Rev 2009;(4):CD000028.

45. Beckett NS, Peters R, Fletcher AE, et al. Treatment of hypertension in patients 80 years of age or older. N Engl J Med 2008;358:1887–98.

46. Brugts JJ, Yetgin T, Hoeks SE, et al. The benefits of statins in people without established cardiovascular disease but with cardiovascular risk factors: meta-analysis of randomised controlled trials. BMJ 2009;338:b2376.

47. Manktelow BN, Potter JF. Interventions in the management of serum lipids for preventing stroke recurrence. Cochrane Database Syst Rev 2009;(3):CD002091. DOI:10.1002/14651858.CD002091.

48. McGuinness B, Craig D, Bullock R, et al. Statins for the prevention of dementia. Cochrane Database Syst Rev 2009;(2):CD003160.

49. Hooper L, Summerbell CD, Higgins JPT, et al. Reduced or modified dietary fat for preventing cardiovascular disease. Cochrane Database Syst Rev 2000;(2): CD002137.

50. UK Prospective Diabetes Study (UKPDS) Group. Intensive blood-glucose control with sulphonylureas or insulin compared with conventional treatment and risk of complications in patients with type 2 diabetes (UKPDS 33). Lancet 1998;352: 837–53.

51. Grimley EJ, Areosa SA. Effect of the treatment of Type II diabetes mellitus on the development of cognitive impairment and dementia. Cochrane Database Syst Rev 2003;(1):CD003804.

52. Nelson MR, Reid CM, Ryan P, et al. Self-reported adherence with medication and cardiovascular disease outcomes in the Second Australian National Blood Pressure Study (ANBP2). Med J Aust 2006;185:487–9.

Healthy Brain Aging: Effect of Head Injury, Alcohol and Environmental Toxins

Vikas Kumar, MD, PhD, Laurence J. Kinsella, MD*

KEYWORDS

• Cognitive dysfunction • Dementia • Alzheimer's disease

Head injury has been recognized as an increasingly important determinant of late-life cognitive function. Despite a large number of research and clinical studies, no direct link has been established between minor head trauma with or without loss of consciousness and the development of dementia of the Alzheimer type. Similarly for alcohol, low doses have been found to be somewhat protective against dementia, whereas large doses increased the risk of late-life cognitive dysfunction. Among the many environmental toxins suspected of causing cognitive dysfunction, lead intoxication has the strongest evidence to support a link. Cognitive dysfunction may occur due to multiple mechanisms, some listed in **Table 1**.

Traumatic brain injury (TBI) has received a great deal of attention in the popular press. Bob Woodruff, a TV news anchor of the American Broadcasting Corporation suffered severe head trauma from an improvised explosive device (IED) in Iraq in January 2006. His story and his remarkable recovery have been well publicized (http://remind.org/, http://en.wikipedia.org/wiki/Bob_Woodruff). TBI is defined as an insult to the brain from some externally inflicted trauma to the head that results in significant impairment to an individual's physical, psychosocial, and/or cognitive functional abilities.

The Department of Defense has recently initiated a large-scale survey of all enlisted service men and women to determine the frequency of head injury and has found a significant proportion reporting some form of head injury on discharge from service. Despite this, many questions remain regarding the methods used to acquire these data, which are based largely on self-reports of injury. This finding is subject to recall bias and selection bias and poses difficulties in analyzing these data in the years ahead as suggested by Hoge and colleagues.[1]

Department of Neurology and Psychiatry, Saint Louis University, St Louis, MO, USA
* Corresponding author.
E-mail address: laurence.kinsella@fphstl.com (L.J. Kinsella).

Clin Geriatr Med 26 (2010) 29–44
doi:10.1016/j.cger.2009.12.006   **geriatric.theclinics.com**
0749-0690/10/$ – see front matter © 2010 Elsevier Inc. All rights reserved.

Table 1
Proposed mechanisms of brain injury from trauma, alcohol, and environmental toxins

Type of Injury	Potential Mechanisms of Brain Damage
Head injury	- Physical trauma (blunt force, penetrating, shearing) - Diffuse axonal injury - Ischemic injury - Cerebral hypoxia - Cerebral edema - Damage to blood-brain barrier - Neurotransmitter (NMDA receptor and glutamate dependent) excitotoxicity - Cytokine/chemokine injury - Cholinergic dysfunction
Alcohol	- Concussion - Regional brain atrophy (cerebellar hemisphere, vermis, thalamus, pons, and prefrontal cortex, temporal lobe including hippocampus) - Impaired cerebral vasoreactivity - Oxidative stress - Loss of white matter/demyelination
Environmental toxins	- Blood-brain barrier changes - Excitotoxic neuronal injury - Interaction with apoptosis - Alterations in glucose metabolism - Oxidative stress injuries - DNA damage - Proinflammatory cytokine activation - Lipid peroxidation

HEAD INJURY AND RISK FOR DEMENTIA

TBI affects 1.5 to 2 million individuals annually, accounting for 235,000 hospitalizations.[2] The male to female ratio is 2.5 to 1. Sixty-six percent of head injuries occur in those younger than 30 years of age. The annual incidence of TBI is 538 per 100,000; 3% are severe, 6% moderate, and 91% are mild. The Centers for Disease Control and Prevention estimates that approximately 5.3 million Americans live with the effects of TBI. The direct medical costs for treatment of TBI have been estimated at more than $60 billion annually (http://www.cdc.gov/NCIPC/tbi/FactSheets/Facts_About_TBI.pdf).

Risk factors include urban and social deprivation, poor academic performance, poor social or vocational backgrounds, a previous history of TBI, a history of drug and alcohol abuse, and a history of criminal activity and psychopathology.[2,3] The sources of TBI include falls in 32%, motor vehicle accidents in 19%, those who are struck on the head 18%, 10% assault, 11% other, and 10% unknown.[2] Head injury may be penetrating or nonpenetrating.

Several clinical questions were proposed to evaluate the effects of head trauma, alcohol, and environmental toxins on late-life dementia. These include the following:

1. Is head trauma a risk factor for dementia in later life?
2. How severe must the injury be to confer risk?
3. Is alcohol consumption a risk factor for dementia?
4. If so, how much?
5. Is there a dose-response curve for trauma and alcohol?

6. Is there a cause-effect relationship between environmental toxins and the development of dementia?

The literature was reviewed and classified using the American Academy of Neurology (AAN) guidelines for the analysis of scientific merit (AAN Guidelines, http://www.aan.com/guidelines). A Medline search for clinical trials, meta-analyses, and original articles using "head trauma," "traumatic brain injury," "alcohol," "dementia," "cognitive impairment," "prognosis," "toxin," and others was performed. There were 50,922 articles found for TBI, 14,784 articles for alcohol and dementia, 1414 articles for TBI and dementia, and 492 articles for toxin and dementia. The references, reviews and meta-analyses were also screened for additional articles. The articles were classified by strength of data using the AAN guidelines for data analyses.

There are 4 levels of evidence used when analyzing epidemiologic studies. Class I studies are prospective cohort studies that fulfill 4 criteria:

A. The group studied is representative of the population of interest
B. Risk factors are clearly defined and measured
C. Groups matched have no confounding risk factors
D. Association can be expressed as a risk or rate ratio. The rate ratio is greater than 2, with a lower confidence interval (CI) greater than 1.

If all of these criteria are fulfilled, one can conclude that the risk factor is established as contributing to the outcome. The recommendation is that the risk factor should be avoided.

Class II studies are those that are retrospective cohorts or case-control studies. They satisfy criteria A, B and C and can be expressed as an odds ratio (OR) with CIs. To be considered a high quality class II study, the OR must be greater than 1.5 with a lower CI greater than 1. The conclusion based on a class II study may be that the risk factor is a probable contributor to disease outcome and the recommendation would be that the risk factor avoidance should be considered.

Class III studies are all other cohort or case-control studies. They have a narrow spectrum (ie, looking only at TBI injury victims referred for rehabilitation). The statistical outcome would be stated as a group mean with a standard deviation (SD) and *P* values. From this, one could conclude only that the risk factor is a possible contributor, and the recommendations would be that risk avoidance may be considered.

Class IV studies are those not meeting the criteria mentioned earlier, and these would include noncomparative studies, case series, case reports, and expert opinions. The conclusion is that no causal relationship can be supported, and no other recommendation can be made.

In 2008, the Institute of Medicine reported on the risk of dementia after TBI.[4] Following the review of extensive literature in this regard, they concluded that there is sufficient evidence of an association between moderate or severe head trauma and dementia of the Alzheimer type. There is limited evidence of an association between mild TBI with loss of consciousness and dementia, and there is inadequate evidence of an association between mild TBI without loss of consciousness and dementia.

Among the strongest class I articles, Plassman and colleagues[5] performed a prospective historical cohort study on 548 World War II veterans with a documented history of nonpenetrating head trauma versus 1228 patients without head trauma. All were screened for dementia in later life. This screening involved a 3-step process including telephone, Mini-Mental status examination, personal interviews, and neuro-psychological testing.[5]

Head injury was considered mild if there was brief loss of consciousness or post-traumatic amnesia less than 30 minutes, without skull fracture. Moderate head trauma was defined as loss of consciousness of posttraumatic amnesia more than 30 minutes but less than 24 hours without skull fracture. Severe head trauma was defined as those with loss of consciousness or posttraumatic amnesia longer than 24 hours.

The hazard ratio (HR) for the severity of head injury and Alzheimer's disease (AD) and all types of dementia correlated closely. The HR was less than 1 for mild head injury, 2.4 for moderate head injuries, and 4.5 for severe head injury. Similarly, for all types of dementia, the HR for mild head injury was slightly greater than 1, for moderate head injury it was 2.5, and for severe head injury it was 4.5. Overall HRs of 2.0 for AD and 2.2 for dementia were found. Severe TBI increases the risk of AD by a factor of 4.51 (CI 1.77–11.47). Moderate TBI increased the risk of AD by 2.32 (CI 1.04–5.17). There was no increase in risk of dementia for mild TBI (HR 0.76). Based on 1 class I and 9 class II/III studies with data inclusive to 2005, there was sufficient evidence of an association between moderate and severe TBI and dementia, limited evidence of an association between mild TBI with loss of consciousness and dementia, and insufficient evidence of an association between mild TBI without loss of consciousness and dementia. In a population study by Nemetz and colleagues[6] the observed time from TBI to AD was less than the expected time to onset of AD (median 10 vs 18 years, $P = .015$).

A class IV study recently published describes chronic traumatic encephalopathy (CTE), formerly known as dementia pugilistica, in 5 autopsies of former football players. CTE has long been recognized among boxers, but has only recently been appreciated in other contact sports such as football. Unlike AD, CTE lacks amyloid deposition, but shows prominent neurofibrillary tangles due to the accumulation of tau protein. The symptoms include mood disorders, inattention, irritability, and mild to severe cognitive impairment. Further studies are needed to determine the correlation between the number and severity of concussions and the neuropathologic changes.[7]

The APOE gene, which encodes apoE protein, fulfills fundamental functions in lipid transport and neural tissue repair after injury. Apolipoprotein E 4 (APOe4) isoform status has been linked to the risk of dementia in older adults and possibly to poor clinical outcome after head injury and intracerebral hemorrhage.[8] There are conflicting data regarding the role of ApoE in TBI and cognitive decline. There is no clear association between the e4 status and the risk of dementia after TBI.[9,10] However, the higher frequency of TBI and Apo E4 genotype amongst AD patients confirms the synergistic/modifying link between an environmental trigger and genetic susceptibility in the development of dementia.[11,12] In a class III (case series) study of 30 boxers, Jordan and colleagues[13] suggested that boxers with APOE e4 allele possession suffered worse chronic neurologic deficits than the boxers without the APOE e4 allele (chronic brain injury score: mean ± SD of 3.9 ± 2.3 vs 1.8 ± 1.2; $P<.04$). Nevertheless, the use of ApoE as a genotype marker for risk of neurologic sequel in high-risk group such as athletes involved in contact sport is not a proposed test (http://www.alzforum.org/res/for/journal/transcript.asp?liveID=169).[14]

Animal trauma models, genetically engineered animals, and neuroprotective studies have been used to simulate the effects of human head trauma to analyze the mechanisms of neuronal injury. Some of the proposed mechanisms are N-methyl-D-aspartate sensitive necrosis and caspase-dependent apoptosis[15]; high extracellular potassium and consequently glutamate release leading to abnormal expression of hippocampal synaptic plasticity[3]; increased levels of amyloid β peptide leading to inflammatory and immune response and cell death[16]; increased tumor necrosis factor (TNF) α neuronal expression[17]; lipid peroxidation,[18] and so forth. TBI also initiates a neuroinflammatory cascade characterized by astrocytes and microglia activation leading to increased production of immune mediators including cytokines and chemokines.[19] The cholinergic hypothesis proposes that impairment in attention, memory, and executive functioning may be related to cholinergic dysfunction in patients with TBI.[20] In this regard, use of acetylcholinesterase and antiinflammatory agents could hold therapeutic potential in preventing TBI ill-effects. In animal studies, it has been shown that even mild TBI causes robust white matter axonal degeneration followed by profound apoptotic cell death.[21] In terms of gross pathology, diffuse axonal injury (DAI) is a primary feature of head trauma. Future advancements in the diagnosis of brain injury using advanced neuroimaging, such as diffusion tensor imaging (DTI), to delineate the extent of cerebral damage may provide distinctive insight into the temporal pathophysiology and cellular integrity of the brain.

ALCOHOL AND HEALTHY AGING BRAIN

A possible role of lifestyle-related factors has been proposed for age-related cognitive functions. Consumption of chronic alcoholic beverages has been associated with a group of neuropsychiatric symptoms including acute confusional state, cognitive decline, alcohol-related dementia, Wernicke-Korsakoff syndrome, cerebellar degeneration, and Marchiafava Bignami disease.[22] However, moderate alcohol intake has been proposed to be a protective factor against cognitive decline and dementia in several longitudinal studies.[23–25] It may also be protective in head trauma.

With an increase in the older population and the number of people with dementia, identifying alcohol and other potential social factors has importance in determining their protective or causative roles in cognitive function. Salim and colleagues[26] studied a total of 38,019 patients with severe TBI to investigate the relationship between mortality and ethanol. Ethanol-positive patients were younger, had a lower injury severity score, and Glasgow Coma Scale score compared with their ethanol-negative counterparts. Ethanol was associated with reduced mortality (adjusted OR, 0.88; 95% CI, 0.80–0.96; $P = .005$) but higher complications (adjusted OR, 1.24; 95% CI, 1.15–1.33; $P<.001$). This study concluded that serum ethanol is independently associated with decreased mortality in patients with moderate to severe head injuries. However, the study also found that drinkers suffered more complications and more severe injuries than nondrinkers, even though the overall survival rate was higher.[26] Also there is a social change in the use of alcohol among the geriatric population. Recently Blazer and colleagues[27] showed a worrying level of binge drinking among those aged 50 to 64 years. Nineteen percent of men and 13% of women had 2 or more drinks per day, considered heavy or at-risk drinking under American Geriatric Society guidelines for older people. The survey also noted binge drinking in those more than 65 years of age: 14% of men and 3% of women.[27]

There is no single definition of moderate drinking. According to the *Dietary Guidelines for Americans*, drinking in moderation is defined as having no more than 1 drink per day for women and no more than 2 drinks per day for men. This definition refers to the amount consumed on any single day and is not intended as an average over several days, and describes a lower risk pattern of drinking (http://www.health.gov/DIETARYGUIDELINES/dga2005/document/html/chapter9.htm).

Several reports have suggested a J- or U-shaped relationship between alcohol consumption and cognitive impairment, with low levels of consumption having better outcomes than abstainers/moderate-heavy drinkers. In this review the authors discuss some of these longitudinal studies. Readers are also referred to a recent systematic review of alcohol and dementia by Peters and colleagues.[28] In this meta-analyses review, which identified 23 studies (20 epidemiologic cohort, 3 retrospective matched cases and controls nested in a cohort), it was shown that small amounts of alcohol may be protective against dementia and AD but not for vascular dementia or cognitive decline. There is relative risk (RR) reduction mortality for those drinking between 1.5 and 3.5 alcoholic beverages per day. The risk is higher for those who do not consume at all and for those who consume more than 4 standard daily drinks.[29] In this study, abstaining women had a RR of 1.29 (95% CI 1.17–1.42) compared with light drinkers (1–6 drinks per week), whereas the RR for abstaining men was 1.22 (95% CI 1.08–1.37) compared with light drinkers. Heavy-drinking women (>28 drinks per week) had an RR of 1.23 (95% CI 0.85–1.78) and heavy-drinking men (more than 69 drinks per week) had an RR of 2.11 (95% CI 1.66–2.69), both compared with light drinkers. When examining the effects of alcohol consumption and dementia, Solfrizzi and colleagues[30] examined the multivariate HR mild cognitive impairment (MCI) among noncognitively impaired subjects and their progression to dementia among patients with minimal cognitive impairment. They found HRs less than 1 for drinking 1 or 1 to 2 drinks of alcohol per day.[30] Anttila and colleagues,[23] in a prospective population-based study, reported that alcohol drinking in middle age shows a U-shaped relationship with risk of MCI in old age. In an Italian longitudinal study that followed participants aged 65 to 84 years for 3.5 years to ascertain the incidence of MCI and its progress to dementia, it was concluded that, in patients with MCI, up to 1 drink per day of alcohol or wine may decrease the rate of progression to dementia than in abstainers (HR 0.15, CI 0.03–0.77). They did not find any association between higher levels of drinking ($\geq$1 drink/d) and rate of progression to dementia in patients with MCI versus abstainers. More recently, Xu and colleagues[31] again showed a J-shaped relationship between alcohol consumption and development of dementia in MCI patients using a cohort study of 176 MCI patients followed for 2 years. Lifetime and daily alcohol consumption were assessed using self-report questionnaires and reports from caregivers. Thirty-seven percent of these MCI patients developed dementia during this follow-up period and patients who consumed a total of less than or equal to 300 kg alcohol before MCI diagnosis had less cognitive decline than patients who consumed no or more than 300 kg alcohol ($P<.01$). Huang and colleagues,[32] in a community-based dementia-free cohort study, showed that light-to-moderate alcohol drinking may protect against dementia among older people (adjusted RR of 0.5, 95% CI 0.3–0.7). In Bordeaux (France), a population-based prospective study found that subjects drinking 3 to 4 standard glasses of wine per day (>250 and up to 550 mL), categorized as "moderate drinkers", the adjusted ORs were 0.19 ($P<.01$) and 0.28 ($P<.05$) respectively for development of incident dementia and AD compared with the nondrinkers. However, in the mild drinkers (<1–2 glasses/d) there was negative association only with AD (OR = 0.55, $P<.05$). Also, light-to-moderate drinking was significantly associated with a lower risk of any dementia (HR 0.58, 95% CI 0.38–0.90) and vascular dementia (HR 0.29, 95% CI 0.09–0.93).[33] Luchsinger and colleagues,[34] in a cohort of elderly persons from New York City, examined the association between intake of alcoholic beverages and risk of AD and dementia associated with stroke. Intake of 3 daily servings of wine was associated with a lower risk of AD (HR 0.55, 95% CI 0.34–0.89). Intake of liquor, beer, and total alcohol was not associated with a lower risk of AD.[34] Mehlig and colleagues,[35] in a follow-up of the prospective population study of women in Goteborg (Sweden), showed that wine and spirits displayed opposing associations with dementia. Wine was protective for dementia (HR 0.6, 95% CI 0.4–0.8), and the association was strongest among women who consumed wine only (HR 0.3, 95% CI 0.1–0.8). In contrast, consumption of spirits at baseline was associated with slightly increased risk of dementia (HR 1.5, 95% CI 1.0–2.2).[35] In a case-control study from a sample of a prospective, population-based cohort study of participants aged 65 years and older in the Cardiovascular Health Study group, Mukamal and Rockwood[36] concluded that, compared with abstinence, consumption of 1 to 6 drinks per week is associated with a lower risk of incident dementia among older adults. A trend toward greater odds of dementia was associated with heavier alcohol consumption and was most apparent in men and subjects with an apolipoprotein E epsilon 4 allele.[36] In a large, prospective, population-based study (Rotterdam study) participants aged 55 years and older who did not have dementia at baseline and who had complete data on alcohol consumption were followed for an average of 6 years. Light-to-moderate drinking (1–3 drinks/d) was associated significantly with a lower risk of any dementia (HR 0.58, 95% CI 0.38–0.90) and vascular dementia (HR 0.29, 95% CI 0.09–0.93). There was no evidence that the relationship between alcohol and dementia varied by type of alcoholic drink.[24] A longitudinal cohort study conducted in Dubbo, Australia, by Simons and colleagues,[37] which studied participants aged 60 years or older and followed them for 16 years, showed a 34% lower risk for dementia with any intake of alcohol accompanied by maintenance of physical activity. Thomas and Rockwood,[38] using the Canadian Study of Health and Aging (CSHA), a representative national cohort study of patients 65 years of age or older and followed for 18 months, showed that occurrence of all types of dementia except probable AD and short-term mortality was higher in those with definite or questionable alcohol abuse. In a case-control nested in a cohort study among participants in the third Copenhagen City Heart Study aged 65 years or more, amount and type of alcohol and risk of dementia was studied. Although average weekly total alcohol intake had no significant effect on risk of dementia, monthly and weekly intake of wine was significantly associated with a lower risk of dementia. For beer and spirits, a monthly intake of beer was significantly associated with an increased risk of dementia.[25] Binge drinking has been identified as a risk for dementia based on a single class III study. This study was a nested cohort of 554 Finnish twins who had provided data on alcohol consumption in questionnaire form and were followed for 25 years. Alcohol intake screening was performed in 1975 and 1981 and telephone dementia screening was performed in 2001. Binge drinking was defined as those drinking more than 5 beers or more than 1 bottle of wine at a single sitting per month. The risk ratio was 3.2 (CI 1.2–8.6) for dementia. If there was loss of consciousness after binge drinking more than twice, the risk ratio increased to 10.5 (CI 2.4–4.6).[39] As reviewed earlier, protective effects are more likely with wine consumption.

To summarize, there is no evidence/indication that light-to-moderate alcohol consumption is harmful to cognition. It is not possible to define a specific beneficial level of alcohol intake. The evidence also shows chronic heavy alcohol intake may be associated with dementia. Currently, there is no established treatment of alcohol-related cognitive decline/dementia except for abstinence as the most logical step. As a loose guideline, heavy drinkers should cut back or quit, light-to-moderate drinkers need not change their drinking habits, and abstainers should not necessarily be encouraged to begin drinking.

The mechanisms of alcohol's beneficial and deleterious effects on the brain are poorly understood. Underscoring the molecular evidence is beyond the scope of this review, but readers are recommended to review the book by Brust.[40] Radiologic and pathologic evidence shows some of the findings mentioned earlier. In a population-based sample using magnetic resonance imaging (MRI) to study findings of brain white matter lesions and infarcts, den Heijer and colleagues[41] showed that light-to-moderate intake is associated with a lower prevalence of vascular brain findings than abstention and heavy drinking. In a controlled study of structural brain changes over 5 years in healthy and alcoholic men, Pfefferbaum and colleagues[42] showed that brain volume shrinkage is exaggerated in the prefrontal cortex in normal aging. In alcoholics, however, there is additional loss of the gray matter over the anterior superior temporal lobe.[42] Regional brain measures also show significant volume deficits in the cerebellar hemispheres, vermis, pons, thalamus, and cortical areas mentioned earlier.[43] Also, it has been speculated that there is compromised brain circuitry in the pontocerebellar and cerebellothalamic pathways.[44] Most dementias show predominantly cortical or subcortical patterns. Munro and colleagues[45] and Schmidt and colleagues[46] have argued that alcoholic dementia cannot be classified as cortical or subcortical, demonstrating impairments in executive control (cortical function) and memory tasks (subcortical function). Alcoholics display features of frontotemporal dementia. Brun and Andersson[47] found a consistent pattern of synapse loss in the superior laminae of the frontal cortical area 10 in autopsies of alcoholics. Frontal lobe dysfunction has also been shown using neuropsychological tasks such as trail A+B and digital symbol tasks.[48] Recently, researchers using fMRI to monitor brain activity in 15 abstinent long-term alcoholics revealed decreased activation of amygdale and hippocampal regions important for emotions and memory, illustrating the dysfunction of neural circuitry or regional difference in blood flow caused by chronic alcohol intake.[49]

As intervention studies are not feasible in this area, the present best evidence comes from an overview of longitudinal studies. Many of these studies are limited by cross-sectional design, restriction by age or sex, variability in end point or follow-up period, beverages, drinking patterns, genetic factors, and lifestyle-related variability, inclusion of true abstainers, and others. Besides the inherent methodological problems involved in population-based epidemiologic studies, it is also unclear whether the benefit can be ascribed to alcohol itself or to other constituents specific to wine such as polyphenols. Study of these unknown mechanisms in the future could shed more light on the cause-effect relationship.

HEALTHY AGING BRAIN AND ENVIRONMENTAL TOXINS

Environmental toxins have long been suspected of causing brain damage from developing brains of children to the mature adult brain. A vast array of potential toxins have been identified that can be classified broadly as organic chemicals (carbon monoxide, organophosphates, solvent mixtures, nerve gas, and so forth), metals (lead, mercury, aluminum, arsenic, manganese, and so forth), pharmacologic agents (opioid analgesics, psychomotor stimulants, sedatives, and hypnotics), neurotoxins of animals (such as snakes, spiders, scorpions) and marine animals (such as pufferfish, shellfish, ciguatera fish poisoning), to name only a few.[50] Other classes of compounds such as certain plants and mushrooms, ionizing and nonionizing radiation, food additives, and air pollution have been suspected of causing toxicity in the nervous system.

Several metals have toxic actions on nerve cells and neurobehavioral functioning. Clinical and animal data show that lead and manganese are most toxic to the nervous system.[51] Lead has no known cellular function. Approximately 250,000 children in the United States aged 1 to 5 years have blood lead levels greater than 10 μg/dL, the level at which the Centers for Disease Control (CDC) recommends public health actions be initiated (http://www.cdc.gov/nceh/lead/). Overall, the weight of available evidence supports an inverse association between blood lead levels less than 10 µg/dL and the cognitive function of children (http://www.cdc.gov/nceh/lead/publications/PrevLeadPoisoning.pdf). Lead exposure during childhood results in a durable loss of 5 to 7 points on IQ testing and also results in shortened attention span.[52] However, there are limited data examining lead exposure and cognitive dysfunction in older adults. In 3 independent longitudinal studies, Stewart and Schwartz[53] examined cumulative lead exposure and its effect on cognitive function in organic lead manufacturing workers, inorganic lead workers, and residents with environmental lead exposure. These results suggest that higher lead accumulation in the body is associated with poorer cognitive outcome, lower brain volume, and that the effect is persistent (class III evidence). In 1982, the Lead Occupational Study assessed the cognitive abilities of 288 lead-exposed and 181 nonexposed male workers in eastern Pennsylvania.[54] All the workers were given the Pittsburgh Occupational Exposures Test battery, which measures 5 primary cognitive domains: psychomotor speed, spatial function, executive function, general intelligence, and learning and memory. Lead-exposed workers were found to have an average blood lead level of 40 µg/dL, considerably higher than normal, whereas the unexposed workers had an average blood level of 7.2 µg/dL, which was within normal limits. After controlling for age, education, and income, no differences between exposed and control workers were found on neuropsychologic or psychosocial variables. Dose-response analyses among lead-exposed workers showed that cumulative and current exposures were unrelated to neuropsychologic performance. In 2004, this cohort was reevaluated with 83 of the original lead-exposed workers and 51 of the original nonexposed workers.[55] Blood lead and tibia bone lead (which measures cumulative lead level) levels were determined for this study. During a 22-year follow-up, bone lead levels in exposed workers predicted lower current cognitive performance and cognitive decline. In those aged 55 years and older, higher levels of bone lead predicted poorer cognitive scores, suggesting that older workers are more vulnerable to the long-term effects of lead exposure.

Neurofibrillary tangles and senile plaques have been found in children and primates following lead exposures.[56,57] Graves and colleagues[58] studied occupational exposure to lead and solvents. In a meta-analysis of 11 case-control studies of AD, lead exposure was found in 6.1% in cases and 8.3% in controls (RR of 0.71, 95% CI 0.36–1.41). This meta-analysis fails to support a causative role of lead in AD pathogenesis or aggravation. However, the original studies lacked high-risk occupational populations and comparable unexposed controls. In general, there is a call for caution for people working in occupations such as lead battery manufacturing, semiconductor fabrication, ceramics, welding and soldering, and some construction work, regarding the risk of exposure. However, there are no randomized controlled data to support this. Future prospective studies from these high-risk populations are needed.

A possible link between pesticide exposure and Parkinson disease (PD) has also been found. However, the evidence is conflicting. Increased risk from related factors such as exposure to well-water consumption or rural agriculture living[59] has been found in some studies, whereas a lack of evidence has been found in others.[60] A population-based case-controlled study by Firestone and colleagues[61] using self-reported pesticide exposure concluded that exposure to occupational pesticide and lifelong well-water consumption (OR of 1.81, CI 1.02–3.21) are consistent with PD risk, whereas home-based exposures did not have any significant association. Their results suggest a gradient that parallels occupational exposures (maximum for pesticide worker, OR of 2.07, 95% CI 0.67–6.38; and minimum for dairy worker, OR of 0.88, 95% CI 0.46–1.70). More recently, Costello and colleagues,[62] using another case-control study using California Pesticide Reports data from 1974 to 1989, showed that exposure to a combination of pesticides (maneb and paraquat in this study) increases the PD risk by 75% (95% CI 1.13–2.73). This study also shows that persons younger than 60 years at the time of diagnosis were at higher risk when exposed to either agent alone (OR of 2.27, 95% CI 0.91–5.70) or to both the pesticides together (OR of 4.17, 95% CI 1.15–15.16).

It has been suggested that manganese occupational exposure in miners, metal workers, and welders exposed to welding fumes may increase the risk of PD.[63] A case-control study performed on 12,595 persons employed at Caterpillar Inc plants (1976–2004) did not find any association between welding and PD- or Parkinson-like symptoms.[64] Several other case-control studies have also found no association with occupational exposure to manganese.[65,66] However, it is worth mentioning that manganese has been associated with manganism, which resembles PD. However, distinctions between the 2 have been detailed.[67] New evidence and efforts to search for new toxins have revealed the role of nitrosamines, which is present in processed or preserved foods, as a risk factor in causing AD in animal studies.[68–70]

There are potential mechanisms for PD and amyotrophic lateral sclerosis (ALS) associated with aging with respect to environmental agents including virus, prions, and toxins. Western pacific ALS-PDC is an ALS and parkinsonism dementia complex and is among the most well studied diseases in this category. It is found in native Chamorro from the island of Guam. Heavy exposure to the raw or incompletely detoxified seeds of the cycad plant, which contains cycasin containing BMAA (β-N-methylamino-L-alanine), a neurotoxic nonprotein amino acid, has been implicated in several epidemiologic and animal studies.[71–73] Cyasin may act as a slow toxin that causes postmitotic neurons to undergo slow irreversible degeneration.[74] A vital question is whether these toxins are sufficient in causing neurodegeneration or act as an accelerant of cell death. Animal models have suggested that neurotoxins alone, without genetic cofactors, are sufficient to cause AD, PD, and ALS.[75]

Data linking environmental toxins and dementia are scarce and conflicting. Reanalyses of 11 European Community Concerted Action Epidemiology of Dementia (EURODEM) case-control studies of AD did not find environmental toxins as a significant interacting factor.[76] Hubble and colleagues,[77] in a case-control study using a cohort of 43 patients with PD with dementia and 51 patients with PD without dementia, showed that pesticide exposure in conjunction with genetic factors may play a role in PD with dementia, illustrating the role of gene-toxin interaction. Rondeau and colleagues[78] showed that binding of aluminum to its cofactor and its interaction with aluminum were not significantly associated with the risk of AD. In a case-control study, Tsai and colleagues[79] found that well-water drinking was a risk factor for the development of PD in the young. Stern and colleagues[80] found no relation with well water, exposure to herbicides, pesticides, or industrial toxins and the risk of PD. They analyzed various environmental exposures and early life experiences in 80 patients with old-onset PD (at an age older than 60 years), 69 young-onset patients (age of onset less than 40 years), and 149 age- and sex-matched control subjects. Smoking was inversely associated with PD in their study, which has been shown to be a consistent finding in several other studies.[81,82] The possible mechanism for why smoking may reduce the risk of PD may be that the substances present in cigarette smoke, such as carbon monoxide or nicotine, may exert a protective effect and thus aid in the survival of dopaminergic neurons. Another plausible mechanism is that smoking alters the activity of metabolic enzymes or competes with other substrates, and thus alters the production of toxic endogenous (dopamine quinines) or exogenous metabolites.[83,84] This evidence comes from animal studies. Menegon and colleagues[85] studied the role of glutathione transferase (GST) polymorphisms in the pathogenesis of PD. GST subtypes were genotyped in 95 PD patients and 95 controls using the polymerase chain reaction (PCR). Pesticide exposure was assessed in all patients and controls. The distribution of the GSTP1 genotypes differed significantly between patients and controls, suggesting a genetic susceptibility to PD from pesticides.[85]

There are multiple theories regarding toxins and cognitive dysfunction in the literature. The evidence comes mostly from animal studies or from postmortem studies, and the level of evidence does not favor one more than the other. Subtle changes of the blood-brain barrier[86] secondary to hypertension, age-related ischemia leading to accumulation of neurotoxins, excitotoxic mechanisms leading to accumulation of calcium, increased oxidative stress[87] leading to loss of dopaminergic neurons secondary to posttranslational modifications,[88] interaction with cellular repair mechanisms,[89] increased metal accumulation such as iron[90] and manganese,[91] and inflammation in the brain[92] are some of the plausible theories. Deleterious effects of lead are proposed to be potentially mediated through alterations in glucocorticoid interactions with the mesocorticolimbic dopamine system.[93] Lead exposure has also been hypothesized to cause inhibition of glucose-using enzymes, increasing the risk of cerebral hypometabolism.[94] Calcium and iron have recently been shown to be important in the pathogenesis of dementia. Although they are required for general cellular functions including oxygen transportation, myelin synthesis, neurotransmitter production, and electron transfers, a pathologic increase in their levels favors oxidative stress and mitochondrial damage, leading to neuronal death.[95–97] This is also supported by postmortem observations that patients with AD or PD show a dramatic increase in their brain iron content.

Reviewing the literature for environmental toxins, the authors found several single case reports regarding neurotoxicity potential for an agent. Well-designed epidemiologic studies are lacking, and few conclusions implicating toxins and cognitive decline can be made. Many of the reported epidemiologic studies are inadequate because of lack of proper matching of exposed subjects and unexposed controls for demographic parameters, genetic predisposition, physiologic changes with aging, premorbid cognitive ability, and so forth. A prolonged period of latency between exposure and disease is a significant limitation. The topic is difficult to study because of concurrent or successive exposure to different environmental factors. With well-designed population studies or animal models, the interactions of toxins and the nervous system and a link with cognitive decline may be answerable.

In conclusion, TBI is associated with dementia of the AD type in a dose-dependent fashion. Minor head trauma is poorly associated with dementia. CTE, long recognized among boxers with recurrent moderate TBI, is now being recognized in football players. The association between APOe4 status, AD, and TBI is unsettled. Alcohol is associated with dementia in binge drinkers but is possibly protective at doses of 1 to 3 wine servings per day. The interaction of environmental toxins needs further studies to reach any conclusive pronouncement.

REFERENCES

1. Hoge CW, Goldberg HM, Castro CA. Care of war veterans with mild traumatic brain injury–flawed perspectives. N Engl J Med 2009;360:1588.
2. Rutland-Brown W, Langlois JA, Thomas KE, et al. Incidence of traumatic brain injury in the United States, 2003. J Head Trauma Rehabil 2006;21:544.
3. Albensi BC, Janigro D. Traumatic brain injury and its effects on synaptic plasticity. Brain Inj 2003;17:653.

4. Institute of Medicine. Gulf war and health: volume 7: long-term consequences of traumatic brain injury. Washington, DC: National Academies Press; 2008.

5. Plassman BL, Havlik RJ, Steffens DC, et al. Documented head injury in early adulthood and risk of Alzheimer's disease and other dementias. Neurology 2000;55:1158.

6. Nemetz PN, Leibson C, Naessens JM, et al. Traumatic brain injury and time to onset of Alzheimer's disease: a population-based study. Am J Epidemiol 1999;149:32.

7. McKee AC, Cantu RC, Nowinski CJ, et al. Chronic traumatic encephalopathy in athletes: progressive tauopathy after repetitive head injury. J Neuropathol Exp Neurol 2009;68:709.

8. Tzourio C, Arima H, Harrap S, et al. APOE genotype, ethnicity, and the risk of cerebral hemorrhage. Neurology 2008;70:1322.

9. Rapoport M, Wolf U, Herrmann N, et al. Traumatic brain injury, Apolipoprotein E-epsilon4, and cognition in older adults: a two-year longitudinal study. J Neuropsychiatry Clin Neurosci 2008;20:68.

10. Raymont V, Greathouse A, Reding K, et al. Demographic, structural and genetic predictors of late cognitive decline after penetrating head injury. Brain 2008;131:543.

11. Graham DI, Gentleman SM, Nicoll JA, et al. Is there a genetic basis for the deposition of beta-amyloid after fatal head injury? Cell Mol Neurobiol 1999; 19:19.

12. Mauri M, Sinforiani E, Bono G, et al. Interaction between Apolipoprotein epsilon 4 and traumatic brain injury in patients with Alzheimer's disease and mild cognitive impairment. Funct Neurol 2006;21:223.

13. Jordan BD, Relkin NR, Ravdin LD, et al. Apolipoprotein E epsilon4 associated with chronic traumatic brain injury in boxing. JAMA 1997;278:136.

14. Alzheimer Research Forum Live Discussion: sports concussions, dementia, and ApoE genotyping: what can scientists tell the public? What's up for research? J Alzheimers Dis 2009;16:657.

15. Allen JW, Knoblach SM, Faden AI. Combined mechanical trauma and metabolic impairment in vitro induces NMDA receptor-dependent neuronal cell death and caspase-3-dependent apoptosis. FASEB J 1999;13:1875.

16. Crawford FC, Wood M, Ferguson S, et al. Genomic analysis of response to traumatic brain injury in a mouse model of Alzheimer's disease (APPsw). Brain Res 2007;1185:45.

17. Knoblach SM, Fan L, Faden AI. Early neuronal expression of tumor necrosis factor-alpha after experimental brain injury contributes to neurological impairment. J Neuroimmunol 1999;95:115.

18. Uryu K, Laurer H, McIntosh T, et al. Repetitive mild brain trauma accelerates Abeta deposition, lipid peroxidation, and cognitive impairment in a transgenic mouse model of Alzheimer amyloidosis. J Neurosci 2002;22:446.

19. Lloyd E, Somera-Molina K, Van Eldik LJ, et al. Suppression of acute proinflammatory cytokine and chemokine upregulation by post-injury administration of a novel small molecule improves long-term neurologic outcome in a mouse model of traumatic brain injury. J Neuroinflammation 2008;5:28.

20. Bennouna M, Greene VB, Defranoux L. [Cholinergic hypothesis in psychosis following traumatic brain injury and cholinergic hypothesis in schizophrenia: a link?]. Encephale 2007;33:616.

21. Dikranian K, Cohen R, Mac Donald C, et al. Mild traumatic brain injury to the infant mouse causes robust white matter axonal degeneration which precedes apoptotic death of cortical and thalamic neurons. Exp Neurol 2008;211:551.

22. Kinsella LJ, Riley DE. RD: Nutritional disorders of the nervous system and the effects of alcohol. In: Goetz CG, editor. Textbook of clinical neurology. 3rd edition. Philadelphia: Saunders Elsevier; 2007. p. xvii.
23. Anttila T, Helkala EL, Viitanen M, et al. Alcohol drinking in middle age and subsequent risk of mild cognitive impairment and dementia in old age: a prospective population based study. BMJ 2004;329:539.
24. Ruitenberg A, van Swieten JC, Witteman JC, et al. Alcohol consumption and risk of dementia: the Rotterdam Study. Lancet 2002;359:281.
25. Truelsen T, Thudium D, Gronbaek M. Amount and type of alcohol and risk of dementia: the Copenhagen City Heart Study. Neurology 2002;59:1313.
26. Salim A, Ley EJ, Cryer HG, et al. Positive serum ethanol level and mortality in moderate to severe traumatic brain injury. Arch Surg 2009;144:865.
27. Blazer DG, Wu LT. The epidemiology of substance use and disorders among middle aged and elderly community adults: national survey on drug use and health. Am J Geriatr Psychiatry 2009;17:237.
28. Peters R, Peters J, Warner J, et al. Alcohol, dementia and cognitive decline in the elderly: a systematic review. Age Ageing 2008;37:505.
29. Gronbaek M, Deis A, Becker U, et al. Alcohol and mortality: is there a U-shaped relation in elderly people? Age Ageing 1998;27:739.
30. Solfrizzi V, D'Introno A, Colacicco AM, et al. Alcohol consumption, mild cognitive impairment, and progression to dementia. Neurology 2007;68:1790.
31. Xu G, Liu X, Yin Q, et al. Alcohol consumption and transition of mild cognitive impairment to dementia. Psychiatry Clin Neurosci 2009;63:43.
32. Huang W, Qiu C, Winblad B, et al. Alcohol consumption and incidence of dementia in a community sample aged 75 years and older. J Clin Epidemiol 2002;55:959.
33. Letenneur L. Risk of dementia and alcohol and wine consumption: a review of recent results. Biol Res 2004;37:189.
34. Luchsinger JA, Tang MX, Siddiqui M, et al. Alcohol intake and risk of dementia. J Am Geriatr Soc 2004;52:540.
35. Mehlig K, Skoog I, Guo X, et al. Alcoholic beverages and incidence of dementia: 34-year follow-up of the prospective population study of women in Goteborg. Am J Epidemiol 2008;167:684.
36. Mukamal KJ, Kuller LH, Fitzpatrick AL, et al. Prospective study of alcohol consumption and risk of dementia in older adults. JAMA 2003;289:1405.
37. Simons LA, Simons J, McCallum J, et al. Lifestyle factors and risk of dementia: Dubbo Study of the elderly. Med J Aust 2006;184:68.
38. Thomas VS, Rockwood KJ. Alcohol abuse, cognitive impairment, and mortality among older people. J Am Geriatr Soc 2001;49:415.
39. Jarvenpaa T, Rinne JO, Koskenvuo M, et al. Binge drinking in midlife and dementia risk. Epidemiology 2005;16:766.
40. Brust JCM. Neurological aspects of substance abuse. 2nd edition. Philadelphia: Elsevier; 2004.
41. den Heijer T, Vermeer SE, van Dijk EJ, et al. Alcohol intake in relation to brain magnetic resonance imaging findings in older persons without dementia. Am J Clin Nutr 2004;80:992.
42. Pfefferbaum A, Sullivan EV, Rosenbloom MJ, et al. A controlled study of cortical gray matter and ventricular changes in alcoholic men over a 5-year interval. Arch Gen Psychiatry 1998;55:905.
43. Pfefferbaum A, Lim KO, Zipursky RB, et al. Brain gray and white matter volume loss accelerates with aging in chronic alcoholics: a quantitative MRI study. Alcohol Clin Exp Res 1992;16:1078.

44. Sullivan EV. Compromised pontocerebellar and cerebellothalamocortical systems: speculations on their contributions to cognitive and motor impairment in nonamnesic alcoholism. Alcohol Clin Exp Res 2003;27:1409.

45. Munro CA, Saxton J, Butters MA. Alcohol dementia: "cortical" or "subcortical" dementia? Arch Clin Neuropsychol 2001;16:523.

46. Schmidt KS, Gallo JL, Ferri C, et al. The neuropsychological profile of alcohol-related dementia suggests cortical and subcortical pathology. Dement Geriatr Cogn Disord 2005;20:286.

47. Brun A, Andersson J. Frontal dysfunction and frontal cortical synapse loss in alcoholism–the main cause of alcohol dementia? Dement Geriatr Cogn Disord 2001;12:289.

48. Davies SJ, Pandit SA, Feeney A, et al. Is there cognitive impairment in clinically 'healthy' abstinent alcohol dependence? Alcohol Alcohol 2005;40:498.

49. Marinkovic K, Oscar-Berman M, Urban T, et al. Alcoholism and dampened temporal limbic activation to emotional faces. Alcohol Clin Exp Res 2009;33: 1880–92.

50. Aminoff M, Yuen TS, Schwartz NE. Effects of toxins and physical agents on the nervous system. In: Bradley WG, editor. 5th edition, Neurology in clinical practice, vol. II. Philadelphia: Butterworth-Heinemann/Elsevier; 2008. p. 1709.

51. Shukla GS, Singhal RL. The present status of biological effects of toxic metals in the environment: lead, cadmium, and manganese. Can J Physiol Pharmacol 1984;62:1015.

52. Needleman HL, Gunnoe C, Leviton A, et al. Deficits in psychologic and class-room performance of children with elevated dentine lead levels. N Engl J Med 1979;300:689.

53. Stewart WF, Schwartz BS. Effects of lead on the adult brain: a 15-year exploration. Am J Ind Med 2007;50:729.

54. Parkinson DK, Ryan C, Bromet EJ, et al. A psychiatric epidemiologic study of occupational lead exposure. Am J Epidemiol 1986;123:261.

55. Khalil N, Morrow LA, Needleman H, et al. Association of cumulative lead and neurocognitive function in an occupational cohort. Neuropsychology 2009;23:10.

56. Niklowitz WJ, Mandybur TI. Neurofibrillary changes following childhood lead encephalopathy. J Neuropathol Exp Neurol 1975;34:445.

57. Wu J, Basha MR, Brock B, et al. Alzheimer's disease (AD)-like pathology in aged monkeys after infantile exposure to environmental metal lead (Pb): evidence for a developmental origin and environmental link for AD. J Neurosci 2008;28:3.

58. Graves AB, van Duijn CM, Chandra V, et al. Occupational exposures to solvents and lead as risk factors for Alzheimer's disease: a collaborative re-analysis of case-control studies. EURODEM Risk Factors Research Group. Int J Epidemiol 1991;20(Suppl 2):S58.

59. Koller W, Vetere-Overfield B, Gray C, et al. Environmental risk factors in Parkinson's disease. Neurology 1990;40:1218.

60. Gorell JM, Johnson CC, Rybicki BA, et al. The risk of Parkinson's disease with exposure to pesticides, farming, well water, and rural living. Neurology 1998; 50:1346.

61. Firestone JA, Smith-Weller T, Franklin G, et al. Pesticides and risk of Parkinson disease: a population-based case-control study. Arch Neurol 2005;62:91.

62. Costello S, Cockburn M, Bronstein J, et al. Parkinson's disease and residential exposure to maneb and paraquat from agricultural applications in the central valley of California. Am J Epidemiol 2009;169:919.

63. Santamaria AB, Cushing CA, Antonini JM, et al. State-of-the-science review: Does manganese exposure during welding pose a neurological risk? J Toxicol Environ Health B Crit Rev 2007;10:417.
64. Marsh GM, Gula MJ. Employment as a welder and Parkinson disease among heavy equipment manufacturing workers. J Occup Environ Med 2006;48: 1031.
65. Fall PA, Fredrikson M, Axelson O, et al. Nutritional and occupational factors influencing the risk of Parkinson's disease: a case-control study in southeastern Sweden. Mov Disord 1999;14:28.
66. Seidler A, Hellenbrand W, Robra BP, et al. Possible environmental, occupational, and other etiologic factors for Parkinson's disease: a case-control study in Germany. Neurology 1996;46:1275.
67. Jankovic J. Searching for a relationship between manganese and welding and Parkinson's disease. Neurology 2005;64:2021.
68. de la Monte SM, Neusner A, Chu J, et al. Epidemilogical trends strongly suggest exposures as etiologic agents in the pathogenesis of sporadic Alzheimer's disease, diabetes mellitus, and non-alcoholic steatohepatitis. J Alzheimers Dis 2009;17:519.
69. de la Monte SM, Tong M. Mechanisms of nitrosamine-mediated neurodegeneration: potential relevance to sporadic Alzheimer's disease. J Alzheimers Dis 2009; 17:817–25.
70. de la Monte SM, Neusner A, Chu J, et al. Epidemilogical trends strongly suggest exposures as etiologic agents in the pathogenesis of sporadic Alzheimer's disease, diabetes mellitus, and non-alcoholic steatohepatitis. J Alzheimers Dis 2009;17:519–29.
71. Ly PT, Singh S, Shaw CA. Novel environmental toxins: steryl glycosides as a potential etiological factor for age-related neurodegenerative diseases. J Neurosci Res 2007;85:231.
72. Murch SJ, Cox PA, Banack SA. A mechanism for slow release of biomagnified cyanobacterial neurotoxins and neurodegenerative disease in Guam. Proc Natl Acad Sci U S A 2004;101:12228.
73. Spencer PS, Kisby GE, Ludolph AC. Slow toxins, biologic markers, and long-latency neurodegenerative disease in the western Pacific region. Neurology 1991;41:62.
74. Spencer PS, Ludolph AC, Kisby GE. Neurologic diseases associated with use of plant components with toxic potential. Environ Res 1993;62:106.
75. Shaw CA, Hoglinger GU. Neurodegenerative diseases: neurotoxins as sufficient etiologic agents? Neuromolecular Med 2008;10:1.
76. van Duijn CM, Stijnen T, Hofman A. Risk factors for Alzheimer's disease: overview of the EURODEM collaborative re-analysis of case-control studies. EURODEM Risk Factors Research Group. Int J Epidemiol 1991;20(Suppl 2):S4.
77. Hubble JP, Kurth JH, Glatt SL, et al. Gene-toxin interaction as a putative risk factor for Parkinson's disease with dementia. Neuroepidemiology 1998;17:96.
78. Rondeau V, Iron A, Letenneur L, et al. Analysis of the effect of aluminum in drinking water and transferrin C2 allele on Alzheimer's disease. Eur J Neurol 2006;13:1022.
79. Tsai CH, Lo SK, See LC, et al. Environmental risk factors of young onset Parkinson's disease: a case-control study. Clin Neurol Neurosurg 2002;104:328.
80. Stern M, Dulaney E, Gruber SB, et al. The epidemiology of Parkinson's disease. A case-control study of young-onset and old-onset patients. Arch Neurol 1991;48:903.

81. Kessler II, Diamond EL. Epidemiologic studies of Parkinson's disease. I. Smoking and Parkinson's disease: a survey and explanatory hypothesis. Am J Epidemiol 1971;94:16.

82. Thacker EL, O'Reilly EJ, Weisskopf MG, et al. Temporal relationship between cigarette smoking and risk of Parkinson disease. Neurology 2007;68:764.

83. Quik M. Smoking, nicotine and Parkinson's disease. Trends Neurosci 2004;27:561.

84. Ross GW, Petrovitch H. Current evidence for neuroprotective effects of nicotine and caffeine against Parkinson's disease. Drugs Aging 2001;18:797.

85. Menegon A, Board PG, Blackburn AC, et al. Parkinson's disease, pesticides, and glutathione transferase polymorphisms. Lancet 1998;352:1344.

86. Mooradian AD. Effect of aging on the blood-brain barrier. Neurobiol Aging 1988;9:31.

87. Koziorowski D, Jasztal J. [Factors which can play important role in pathogenesis of Parkinson disease]. Neurol Neurochir Pol 1999;33:907.

88. Danielson SR, Andersen JK. Oxidative and nitrative protein modifications in Parkinson's disease. Free Radic Biol Med 2008;44:1787.

89. Eizirik DL, Spencer P, Kisby GE. Potential role of environmental genotoxic agents in diabetes mellitus and neurodegenerative diseases. Biochem Pharmacol 1996; 51:1585.

90. Enochs WS, Sarna T, Zecca L, et al. The roles of neuromelanin, binding of metal ions, and oxidative cytotoxicity in the pathogenesis of Parkinson's disease: a hypothesis. J Neural Transm Park Dis Dement Sect 1994;7:83.

91. Seth PK, Chandra SV. Neurotransmitters and neurotransmitter receptors in developing and adult rats during manganese poisoning. Neurotoxicology 1984;5:67.

92. Liu B, Gao HM, Wang JY, et al. Role of nitric oxide in inflammation-mediated neurodegeneration. Ann N Y Acad Sci 2002;962:318.

93. White LD, Cory-Slechta DA, Gilbert ME, et al. New and evolving concepts in the neurotoxicology of lead. Toxicol Appl Pharmacol 2007;225:1.

94. Yun SW, Hoyer S. Effects of low-level lead on glycolytic enzymes and pyruvate dehydrogenase of rat brain in vitro: relevance to sporadic Alzheimer's disease? J Neural Transm 2000;107:355.

95. Bermejo F, Vega S, Olazaran J, et al. [Mild cognitive impairment in the elderly]. Rev Clin Esp 1998;198:159.

96. Surmeier DJ. Calcium, ageing, and neuronal vulnerability in Parkinson's disease. Lancet Neurol 2007;6:933.

97. Zecca L, Youdim MB, Riederer P, et al. Iron, brain ageing and neurodegenerative disorders. Nat Rev Neurosci 2004;5:863.

Healthy Brain Aging: What Has Sleep Got To Do With It?

Raman K. Malhotra, MD[a,b,*], Abhilash K. Desai, MD[b,c]

KEYWORDS

- Sleep • Memory • Dementia • Cognition
- Insomnia • Sleep apnea

For centuries, sleep was considered a passive activity, perhaps even a period of time in life that was a hindrance or barrier to getting more things accomplished. Although the exact function of sleep is still being explored, experts now believe it plays a valuable role in maintaining health. Recent research has begun to focus on its importance to cardiovascular health, longevity, mood, and immune function, although ever since scientists began to study sleep, there has been a belief in its vital role in learning, memory, and overall central nervous system homeostasis. Despite new awareness of the consequences of sleep loss, over the past 100 years, the population's total sleep time has diminished. On average, Americans are sleeping 6.8 hours per night, as reported in 2005 (National Sleep Foundation Sleep in America poll[1]). Twenty two percent of Americans believe they are not getting the amount of sleep they need. Whether or not they are deciding to voluntarily deprive themselves of adequate sleep or are not obtaining good quality sleep secondary to a sleep disorder, there is increasing evidence of the immediate and long-term consequences, especially relating to the brain. As described in this article, sleep deprivation and sleep disruption may not only have transient effects on cognition but also result in permanent and long-standing effects on processes of memory and brain plasticity.

Sleep deprivation and sleep disorders are common in the general population. The Institute of Medicine in 2006 estimated that 50 to 70 million Americans chronically suffer from a disorder of sleep or wakefulness, hindering daily functioning.[2] Although many effective treatments for sleep disorders exist, the majority of patients remain

[a] SLUCare Sleep Disorders Center, 3545 Lafayette Avenue, St Louis, MO 63104, USA
[b] Department of Neurology and Psychiatry, Saint Louis University School of Medicine, Monteleone Hall, 1438 South Grand Boulevard, St Louis, MO 63104, USA
[c] Center for Healthy Brain Aging, Monteleone Hall, 1438 South Grand Boulevard, St Louis, MO 63104, USA
* Corresponding author. Department of Neurology and Psychiatry, Saint Louis University School of Medicine, Monteleone Hall, 1438 South Grand Boulevard, St Louis, MO 63104.
E-mail address: rmalhot1@slu.edu (R.K. Malhotra).

Clin Geriatr Med 26 (2010) 45–56
doi:10.1016/j.cger.2009.11.001
0749-0690/10/$ – see front matter © 2010 Elsevier Inc. All rights reserved.

undiagnosed.[3] The most prevalent sleep disorders, such as obstructive sleep apnea (OSA), insomnia, and restless legs syndrome, can cause daytime cognitive impairment. When patients do seek treatment for their sleep disorders, many of the pharmacologic agents available may paradoxically have detrimental effects on cognition and daytime functioning. For these reasons, it has become increasingly important for medical professionals to be able to correctly recognize and appropriately treat sleep disorders in their patients to maximize cognitive function and brain health.

SLEEP AND ITS EFFECT ON COGNITION
Sleep and Memory

Sleep has been implicated in the encoding and consolidation of memory.[4,5] In a group of healthy adults deprived of sleep for 36 hours continuously, significant impairment in retention of new information was evident compared with controls who were not sleep deprived, even in a subgroup that received caffeine to overcome nonspecific effects of lower alertness.[6] Furthermore, the sleep-deprived subjects displayed significantly worse insight into their performance, resulting in lower predictive ability of performance. Inadequate sleep before learning produces bidirectional changes in episodic encoding activity, involving the inability of the medial temporal lobe (the primary center for encoding) to engage normally during learning, combined with potential compensation attempts by prefrontal regions, which in turn may facilitate recruitment of parietal lobe function.[7] Thus, optimal prefrontal function may be necessary for adequate compensatory strategies to overcome encoding problems due to sleep deprivation. For individuals with pre-existing prefrontal lobe dysfunction (eg, individuals with depression or cerebrovascular disease affecting the frontal lobe), the impact of sleep deprivation on memory encoding may be even greater. Sleep deprivation has also been found to markedly impair hippocampal function, and the hippocampus is critical for learning new episodic information.[8]

There is robust, consistent literature demonstrating the need for sleep after learning in the subsequent consolidation and enhancement of implicit memories.[4] Recent research has also revealed a strong beneficial effect of sleep on the consolidation of declarative memory.[9,10] Several studies have suggested a critical role for slow wave sleep (SWS) neurophysiology in the offline consolidation of episodic facts.[11] Memories tested after a night of sleep are significantly more resistant to interference, whereas across a waking day, memories are far more susceptible to interference.[12] Functional imaging (eg, functional MRI) studies contrasting sleep-deprived and well-rested brains provide substantial evidence that sleep is important for optimal cognitive function and learning.[13] One mechanism proposed as underlying these effects on hippocampal-dependent learning tasks is the reactivation of memory representations during SWS and possibly rapid eye movement (REM) sleep.[14,15] Using positron emission tomography scanning, it was shown that daytime learning was initially associated with hippocampal activity and during post-training sleep, there was re-emergence of hippocampal activation, specifically during SWS.[16] Even more interesting was the finding that the amount of SWS reactivation in the hippocampus was proportional to the amount of next-day task improvement, suggesting that this reactivation is associated with offline memory improvement. Thus, during sleep, the brain reactivates brain maps that were activated during the previous day, and these unconscious rehearsals strengthen memory. Research has also indicated that the brain may be selectively rehearsing the more difficult aspects of a task.[17]

Stage 2 non–REM (NREM) sleep (marked by sleep spindles or K-complexes on electroencephalogram) has also been implicated in memory consolidation. Increased spindle density after intensive training on a pursuit motor skill task and increased spindle density after combined training on several simple procedural motor tasks have been reported.[18] The mechanistic benefit of sleep spindles may be related to their faster stimulating frequency, a range suggested as facilitating long-term potentiation, a foundational principal of synaptic strengthening in the brain and essential for memory consolidation.[19]

REM sleep may play an important role in emotional memory processing.[20] Experiences that evoke emotions not only encode more strongly but also seem to persist and even improve over time as the delay between learning and testing increases.[21] A consistent relationship between REM sleep and emotional processing has been identified.[20] Increased activity within limbic and paralimbic structures (including the hippocampus and amygdala) during REM sleep offers the ability for reactivation of previously acquired affective experiences. REM sleep (characterized by dominant theta oscillations within subcortical and cortical nodes) may offer large-scale network cooperation at night, allowing the integration and, as a consequence, greater understanding of recently experienced emotional events in the context of pre-existing neocortically stored semantic memory.[20,22] The process of REM sleep mental activity may aid in the resolution of previous emotional conflict, resulting in improved next-day negative mood.[23]

Sleep and Creativity

Sleep is also involved in the association and integration of new experience into pre-existing networks of knowledge.[20] Research involving naps in infants has shown that sleep allows the reinterpretation of prior experience and supports the ability to detect a general pattern in new information.[24] Human memory integration takes time to develop, requiring slow, offline associative processes.[25] In an elegant study, sleeping after exposure to a problem was found to more than double the likelihood of solving it.[26] Thus, during sleep, the brain may also replay collections of memories to discover patterns and thus help find meaning in what has been learned.

Sleep and Neuroplasticity

Rapidly growing experimental evidence supports the notion that sleep plays an active role in modulating synaptic plasticity in the brain.[27] Several neural level mechanistic models of sleep-dependent neuroplasticity have been described.[20] Emerging evidence has suggested a role for sleep in regulating the synaptic connectivity of the brain, principally the neocortex.[28] There is evidence indicating local sleep-dependent neural pruning by SWS, the goal of which may be to regulate neural architecture at a highly specific anatomic level, mapping onto corresponding locations of memory representation.[29] Thus, SWS selectively downscales synaptic strength back to baseline levels, preventing synaptic overpotentiation, which would result in saturated brain plasticity. In doing so, this rescaling leaves behind more efficient and refined memory representations the next day, affording improved recall.[20] In humans, NREM SWS dominates early in the nigh, and stage N2 (stage 2) and REM sleep prevail later in the night. From a memory consolidation perspective, the predominance of hippocampal-neocortical interaction takes place in the early SWS-rich phase of the night, leaving corticocortical connections on offer for later processing during stage N2 and REM sleep.[20] Such a cooperative mechanism produces a network of stored information that is not only more efficient but also, for those representations remaining, more enhanced. Sleep deprivation inhibits adult neurogenesis possibly by elevating corticosterone.[30] Such a suppression of adult neurogenesis and synaptic plasticity may underlie some of the cognitive deficits associated with prolonged sleep deprivation.

One recent study showed amyloid plaques appeared earlier and more often in the brains of mice with chronic sleep deprivation, proposing one possible link between sleep disruption and subsequent development of dementia.[31]

OBSTRUCTIVE SLEEP APNEA AND THE HEALTHY AGING BRAIN

OSA syndrome is a common sleep disorder that involves repetitive occurrence of partial (hypopnea) or complete (apnea) interruptions in airflow during sleep. During these breathing events, blood oxygen saturation can drop to dangerously low levels, eventually leading to arousals from sleep. OSA syndrome affects up to 2% of middle-aged women and 4% of middle-aged men.[32] The prevalence is higher in geriatric populations[33] and African Americans.[34] Unfortunately, most patients continue to remain undiagnosed and untreated.[3] OSA frequently causes neurocognitive decline and has been associated with long-term cardiovascular consequences, both of which may make the brain more vulnerable to other insults (eg, neurodegenerative processes).

Cognitive Deficits Associated with Obstructive Sleep Apnea

Clinical symptoms of OSA include not only daytime sleepiness but also a variety of cognitive complaints that are similar to those seen in the early stages of dementing illnesses.[35] There are many studies published on the neuropsychologic effects of OSA, including comparisons with age-matched controls or normative data of the general population. Treatment of OSA, with continuous positive airway pressure (CPAP) or other effective treatments (surgery), has been shown to improve these neuropsychologic deficits, although these studies are limited by confounders, such as comorbid medical conditions and age-related effects.[35] A comprehensive literature review[35] and one meta-analysis[36] affirm that OSA has substantial effects on attention and vigilance. Specifically, patients with OSA struggle with sustained attention, and performance worsens as the duration of the task lengthens.[37] In addition, OSA patients seem to perform poorly on tests of executive function. These include difficulties with planning, sequential thinking, and constructional ability.[38] Some studies have shown decreases in overall intelligence and language.[36] Although inconsistent, several studies have shown OSA is associated with memory difficulties.[39,40] There also seems to be a significant, although small, association between polysomnographic measures of sleep apnea and working and declarative memory.[41]

The precise mechanism of how OSA causes its symptoms is unclear, but most investigators agree the culprit is likely intermittent sleep-related hypoxemia and repetitive cortical arousals from sleep. This chronic sleep fragmentation and hypoxemia that results from OSA may alter the restorative process that normally occurs during sleep. This disruption of cellular and chemical homeostasis may create a chain reaction that leads to altered neuronal and glial viability.[35] Animal models of sleep apnea show increased neuronal apoptosis in the hippocampus and overlying cortical region.[42] Further proof of this relationship includes human studies that have found a relationship between degree of hypoxemia, frequency of respiratory events (measured by an apnea-hypopnea index), and resulting cognitive dysfunction. The majority of studies have found a significant association between apnea severity and at least one domain of cognitive performance. Hypoxemia seems more associated with performance on tests of global cognitive functioning, whereas measures of sleep fragmentation and arousal are associated with performance on tests of attention and vigilance.[35]

Treatment of Obstructive Sleep Apnea

CPAP is the treatment of choice for most adult patients with OSA.[43] CPAP provides air pressure to the upper airway, preventing it from collapsing during sleep, thus preventing the hypoxemia and sleep fragmentation normally associated with sleep apnea. CPAP improves many of the neurocognitive deficits seen in OSA, although not entirely. Improvements in different neuropsychologic domains have been noted with treatment of sleep apnea with both CPAP and surgical treatments for sleep apnea.[35]

OSA has been found to aggravate cognitive dysfunction in dementia and thus may be a reversible cause of cognitive loss in patients with Alzheimer's disease.[44] CPAP reduces subjective daytime sleepiness in patients with Alzheimer's disease and OSA.[45] One recent small study has shown slowing of cognitive deterioration in Alzheimer's dementia patients with OSA who were able to use CPAP as compared with the ones who were not.[46]

Permanent Central Nervous System Injury in Obstructive Sleep Apnea

Alternatively, many sleep apnea patients, despite adequate treatment, are left with residual neurocognitive deficits.[47,48] This has led to speculation that OSA may lead to permanent injury of the central nervous system. Evidence of this lasting damage is supported by studies that have revealed changes in the brains of OSA patients using a variety of imaging modalities. Macey and colleagues,[49] in 2002, published findings showing gray matter loss in the frontal cortex, parietal cortex, temporal lobe, anterior cingulate, and hippocampus of OSA patients on MRI. Several studies have demonstrated hippocampal loss and atrophy in OSA patients[50] on MRI. Magnetic resonance spectroscopy displayed metabolic changes in the brain as compared with control subjects, even after treatment with CPAP.[51] Diffusion tensor imaging showed white matter was affected in OSA patients, specifically in the limbic system, cortex, and the projections to and from the cerebellum.[52] Ficker and colleagues[53] exhibited differences in cerebral perfusion in OSA patients with the use of single-photon emission CT. Kumar and colleagues[54] found that mammillary body volume size was smaller in OSA patients as compared with controls. The mammillary body plays an important role in cognition, as evidenced by other disorders that can affect it, such as Korsakoff's syndrome.

OSA has been shown to be a risk factor for stroke.[55,56] Prestroke white matter changes were seen more commonly in OSA patients and predicted the occurrence of more white matter changes with time.[57] The pathophysiology of this correlation may relate to apneas causing cardiac arrhythmias during sleep, hypoxemia, increased autonomic arousal, elevated catecholamines, and abrupt shifts in cerebral blood flow that occur with repetitive obstructive events and arousals during sleep. OSA has also been found to increase fibrinogen levels,[58] platelet aggregation,[59] and carotid wall thickness[60] and to lead to hypercoagulability,[61] all of which can lead to higher rates of cerebrovascular disease. Through some or all of these mechanisms, this higher risk of stroke in OSA patients may translate into higher rates of vascular dementia in patients with OSA.[62]

SLEEP AND SLEEP DISORDERS IN THE ELDERLY

Other sleep disorders, not only OSA, can cause similar symptoms of cognitive impairment. Insomnia, restless legs syndrome, and circadian rhythm disorders are all common, especially in the elderly. These disorders can be difficult to identify because it can be challenging to distinguish between "normal" aging versus a separate sleep disorder or pathology. It is true that with age, sleep quality and patterns can change.

These changes are gradual over a lifetime. The percentage of SWS (or delta sleep) that a person has at night decreases with age, especially for men.[63] The elderly (over age 65) also have more awakenings during sleep.[64] This leads to older adults being significantly sleepier than younger adults when measured objectively.[65] Despite these changes with age, sleep need remains the same throughout adulthood. Sleep complaints are more common in the elderly, partly due to more comorbid psychiatric and medical conditions that disrupt sleep and concomitantly affect cognition.

COGNITIVE IMPAIRMENT/IMPROVEMENT FROM MEDICATIONS USED FOR SLEEP

Table 1 lists commonly used hypnotics, their potential risks, and safer alternatives. Drugs commonly used to treat insomnia (eg, benzodiazepines and drugs with high anticholinergic properties, such as diphenydramine) have a particularly high risk of cognitive impairment in older adults.[66,67] The risk of hypnotic medication-induced cognitive impairment may be minimized by several strategies, including avoidance of unnecessary medications; use of nonpharmacologic insomnia treatments, such as cognitive-behavioral therapy; and selection of hypnotics least likely to cause cognitive impairment.[67] In people over age 60, the benefits of sedative hypnotics (eg, improvements in sleep latency and total sleep time) may not justify the increased risk, particularly if patients have additional risk factors for cognitive or psychomotor adverse events.[68] Based on limited data, zolpidem, zaleplon, eszopiclone, and ramelteon represent modestly effective and generally well-tolerated treatments for insomnia in older adults.[69] The 2005 National Institutes of Health State-of-the-Science Conference on Insomnia concluded there is no systematic evidence for the effectiveness of many medications, including antihistamines, antidepressants, antipsychotics, and anticonvulsants used off label for the treatment of insomnia, and warned that the risks of use outweighed the benefits.[70] Trazodone, a frequently prescribed antidepressant for insomnia in older persons, is sedating but can cause orthostasis and has no published evidence of sustained efficacy.[71] Benzodiazepine receptor agonists (eg,

Table 1
Commonly used hypnotics in older adults, their potential risks, and suggested safer alternatives

Drugs	Indication	Safe Alternatives	Concern
Diphenhydramine	Insomnia	Nondrug interventions, BRA, MRA	CI, DS
Trazodone	Insomnia	Nondrug interventions, BRA, MRA	Orthostasis, DS
Flurazepam	Insomnia	Nondrug interventions, BRA, MRA	DS, falls, CI
Quazepam	Insomnia	Nondrug interventions, BRA, MRA	DS, falls, CI
Estazolam	Insomnia	Nondrug interventions, BRA, MRA	DS, falls, CI
Temazepam	Insomnia	Nondrug interventions, BRA, MRA	Falls, CI
Triazolam	Insomnia	Nondrug interventions, BRA, MRA	Falls, CI
Eszopiclone	Insomnia	Nondrug interventions, MRA	Falls
Zolpidem	Insomnia	Nondrug interventions	Falls
Zaleplon	Insomnia	Nondrug interventions	Falls
Ramelteon	Insomnia	Nondrug interventions	Not well studied in older adults

Abbreviations: BRA, benzodiazepine receptor agonists (eg, eszopiclone, zolpidem, and zaleplon), also called nonbenzodiazepine hypnotics; CI, cognitive impairment; DS, daytime sleepiness; MRA, melatonin receptor agonists (eg, ramelteon).

zolpidem, zaleplon, and eszopiclone) have lower frequency of adverse effects (eg, falls and cognitive impairment) than those found in the older benzodiazepines approved as hypnotics (eg, triazolam and temazepam) and thus are preferable for use in older adults in whom short-term therapy of hypnotics is indicated for treatment of insomnia (NIH 2005). In the adult nonelderly population, use of melatonin agonist ramelteon has not been found to be associated with adverse cognitive effects,[72] although it is only effective for sleep onset and not maintenance insomnia. Ramelteon has not been well studied in geriatric populations, although one study did show there was less balance difficulty in the middle of the night in the elderly with use of ramelteon as compared with zolpidem.[73] **Table 2** lists some practical rules to follow when prescribing sedative hypnotics to older individuals for insomnia.

Treatment of excessive daytime sleepiness associated with sleep disorders, such as OSA and narcolepsy, may be treated with modafinil, armodafinil, or stimulants (methylphenidate, D-amphetamines, methamphetamines, or amphetamines). These drugs may also be useful for treatment of idiopathic hypersomnia, hypersomnia related to medications (eg, opioids), and hypersomnia due to a medical condition.[71] These wake-promoting drugs may improve cognitive performance by reducing daytime sleepiness and improving daytime alertness.[71,74,75] **(Table 3)**.

RESEARCH GAPS

Despite the explosion of research recently on the effects of sleep disorders on cognition and the healthy aging brain, many significant questions remain. Much of the current data on sleep and memory are in younger adults and have not included the elderly. Some of the findings in younger subjects (eg, increase in sleep spindle density after motor learning) may not be seen in older adults.[76] It will also be crucial to learn if there is a particular stage of sleep (eg, SWS) that is more important than other stages of sleep in memory processing or influencing cognitive function. Finding this vital piece of information would assist in developing treatments targeting this stage of sleep. Mechanisms linking sleep disorders (eg, OSA) to cognitive impairment in older adults need to be better characterized and identified, especially if they are leading to permanent central nervous system damage. There needs to be more research showing that

---

Table 2
Basic principles in pharmacologic treatment of insomnia

1. After a thorough assessment, establish a clear diagnosis of insomnia by differentiating it from specific sleep disorders causing insomnia, such as restless legs syndrome, REM sleep behavior disorder, or OSA.
2. Consider discontinuing unnecessary medications, medications that are inappropriate for use in the older individual, and medications that may be contributing to insomnia (eg, stimulants).
3. Encourage evidenced-based effective nondrug interventions to treat insomnia, such as cognitive behavioral therapy for insomnia.
4. Take into account chronic conditions leading to cognitive impairment, balance and gait difficulties.
5. Take into account concomitant prescriptions of central nervous system active agents (especially psychotropics and anticholinergic drugs) that may increase the risk of cognitive toxicity that may occur with use of sedative hypnotics.
6. Discuss risks and benefits of sedative hypnotics thoroughly.
7. Start low (eg, half the recommended adult dosage) and go slow (slower titration to final lowest possible therapeutic dose).

Table 3		
Potential cognition-improving drugs used for sleep disorders		
Drugs	**Indication**	**Comment**
Modafinil	EDS due to narcolepsy EDS despite treated OSA EDS due to shift work disorder Idiopathic insomnia Medication-induced hypersomnia	May improve alertness and cognition
Armodafinil	EDS due to narcolepsy EDS despite treated OSA EDS due to shift work disorder	May improve alertness and cognition
Stimulants[a]	Narcolepsy Medication-induced hypersomnia	May improve alertness and cognition

Abbreviation: EDS, excessive daytime sleepiness.
[a] Methylphenidate and amphetamine derivatives.

treating sleep disorders leads to improved cognitive function or halting cognitive decline in patients with progressive dementia. Comparative pharmacovigilance studies focusing on the impact of different sedative hypnotics on cognition are needed, including a better understanding of the risks involved with these medications in the elderly.

SUMMARY

Sleep may have a crucial role in molecular, cellular, and systems-level processes that convert initial, labile memory representations into more permanent ones that are available for continued reactivation and recall over extended periods of time.[77] Optimal sleep before learning is necessary to prepare key neural structures for efficient next-day learning. Without adequate sleep, hippocampal function becomes markedly disrupted, resulting in a decreased ability for recording new experiences, the extent of which seems to be further governed by alterations in prefrontal encoding dynamics. Sleep also protects memory from being lost due to interference (ie, learning disruption). Besides memory, sleep has a role in problem solving, creativity, and regulating emotional brain reactivity.[20] The final goal of sleep-dependent memory processing may be integration of memories into a common schema and thus facilitation of the development of universal concepts, a process that forms the basis of generalized knowledge and creativity.

Assessing the quality of a person's sleep is frequently overlooked during routine physician visits. Many common sleep disorders continue to remain undiagnosed, although they have been associated with neurocognitive dysfunction and frequently respond to treatment. Permanent brain changes may result from sleep disorders, such as OSA, as evidenced by many imaging modalities. It is time for all health care providers to wake up and routinely assess sleep quality and duration in their patients. This is especially important in assessing adults who complain of new-onset memory and cognitive problems.

REFERENCES

1. National Sleep Foundation. Sleep in America Poll 2005. Washington, DC. Available at: http://www.sleepfoundation.org/sites/default/files/2005_summary_of_findings.pdf.

2. Colten HR, Altevogt BM. Sleep disorders and sleep deprivation: an unmet public health problem. Washington, DC: National Academies Press; 2006.
3. Young T, Evans L, Finn L, et al. Estimation of the clinically diagnosed proportion of sleep apnea syndrome in middle-aged men and women. Sleep 1997;20:705–6.
4. Walker MP, Stickgold R. Sleep, memory and plasticity. Annu Rev Psychol 2006; 10:139–66.
5. Stickgold R. Sleep-dependent memory consolidation. Nature 2005;437:1272–8.
6. Harrison Y, Horne JA. Sleep loss and temporal memory. Q J Exp Psychol 2000; 53:271–9.
7. Drummond SP, Brown GG. The effects of total sleep deprivation on cerebral responses to cognitive performance. Neuropsychopharmacology 2001;25: S68–73.
8. Yoo SS, Gujar N, Hu P, et al. The human emotional brain without sleep— a prefrontal amygdala disconnect. Curr Biol 2007;17:R877–8.
9. Stickgold R, James L, Hobson JA. Visual discrimination learning requires sleep after training. Nat Neurosci 2000;3(12):1237–8.
10. Marshall L, Born J. The contribution of sleep to hippocampus-dependent memory consolidation. Trends Cogn Sci 2007;11:442–50.
11. Marshall L, Helgadottir H, Molle M, et al. Boosting slow oscillations during sleep potentiates memory. Nature 2006;444:610–3.
12. Ellenbogen JM, Hulbert JC, Stickgold R. Interfering with theories of sleep and memory: sleep, declarative memory, and associative interference. Curr Biol 2006;16:1290–4.
13. Chee MW, Chuah LY. Functional neuroimaging insights into how sleep and sleep deprivation affect memory and cognition. Curr Opin Neurol 2008;21(4): 417–23.
14. Wilson MA, McNaughton BL. Reactivation of hippocampal ensemble memories during sleep. Science 1994;265:676–9.
15. Ji D, Wilson MA. Coordinated memory replay in the visual cortex and hippocampus during sleep. Nat Neurosci 2007;10:100–7.
16. Peigneux P, Laureys S, Fuchs S, et al. Are spatial memories strengthened in the human hippocampus during slow wave sleep? Neuron 2004;44:535–45.
17. Stickgold R, Ellenbogen JM. Quiet! Sleeping brain at work. Sci Am Mind 2008; 19(4):23–30.
18. Fogel SM, Smith CT. Learning-dependent changes in sleep spindles and Stage 2 sleep. J Sleep Res 2006;15:250–5.
19. Smith CT, Aubrey JB, Peters KR. Different roles for REM and stage 2 sleep in motor learning: a proposed model. Psychologica Belgica 2004;44:81–104.
20. Walker MP. The role of sleep in cognition and emotion. Ann N Y Acad Sci 2009; 1156:168–97.
21. Sharot T, Phelps EA. How arousal modulates memory: disentangling the effects of attention and retention. Cogn Affect Behav Neurosci 2004;4:294–306.
22. Pace-Schott EF, Hobson JA. The neurobiology of sleep: genetics, cellular physiology and subcortical networks. Nat Rev Neurosci 2002;3:591–605.
23. Cartwright R, Agargun MY, Kirkby J, et al. Relation of dreams to waking concerns. Psychiatry Res 2006;141:261–70.
24. Gomez RL, Bootzin RR, Nadel L. Naps promote abstraction in language-learning infants. Psychol Sci 2006;17:670–4.
25. Ellenbogen J, Hu P, Payne JD, et al. Human relational memory requires time and sleep. Proc Natl Acad Sci U S A 2007;104:7723–8.
26. Wagner U, Gais S, Haider H, et al. Sleep inspires insight. Nature 2004;427:352–5.

27. Miyamoto H, Hensch T. Bidirectional interaction of sleep and synaptic plasticity: a view from visual cortex. Sleep Biol Rhythm 2006;4(1):35–43.
28. Tononi G, Cirelli C. Sleep function and synaptic homeostasis. Sleep Med Rev 2006;10:49–62.
29. Huber R, Ghilardi MF, Massimini M, et al. Local sleep and learning. Neuron 2004; 430:78–81.
30. Mirescu C, Peters JD, Noiman L, et al. Sleep deprivation inhibits adult neurogenesis in the hippocampus by elevating glucocorticoids. Proc Natl Acad Sci U S A 2006;103(50):19170–5.
31. Kang JE, Lim MM, Bateman RJ, et al. Amyloid beta dynamics are regulated by orexin and the sleep-wake cycle. Science 2009. [Epub ahead of print].
32. Young T, Dempsey J, Skatrud J, et al. The occurrence of sleep-disordered breathing among middle-aged adults. N Engl J Med 1993;328:1230–5.
33. Ancoli-Israel S, Kripke DF, Klauer MR, et al. Sleep-disordered breathing in community dwelling elderly. Sleep 2001;14(6):486–95.
34. Redline S, Tishler PV, Hans MG, et al. Racial differences in sleep-disordered breathing in African-Americans and Caucasians. Am J Respir Crit Care Med 1997;155(5):1820.
35. Aloia MS, Arnedt JT, Davis JD, et al. Neuropsychological sequelae of obstructive sleep apnea-hyopnea syndrome: a critical review. J Int Neuropsychol Soc 2004; 10(5):772–85.
36. Beebe DW, Groesz L, Wells C, et al. The neuropsychological effects of obstructive sleep apnea: a meta-analysis of norm-referenced and case-controlled data. Sleep 2003;26(3):298–307.
37. Weaver TE. Outcome measurement in sleep medicine practice and research. Part 2: assessment of neurobehavioral performance and mood. Sleep med Rev 2001;5(3):223–36.
38. Sateia MJ. Neuropsycological impairment and quality of life in obstructive sleep apnea. Clin Chest Med 2003;24(2):249–59.
39. Findley LJ, Barth JT, Powers DC, et al. Cognitive impairment in patients with obstructive sleep apnea and associated hypoxemia. Chest 1986;90(5): 686–90.
40. Bedard MA, Montplaisir J, Richer F, et al. Obstructive sleep apnea syndrome: pathogenesis of neuropsychological deficits. J Clin Exp Neuropsychol 1991; 13(6):950–64.
41. Adams N, Strauss M, Schluchter M, et al. Relation of measures of sleep-disordered breathing to neuropsychological functioning. Am J Respir Crit Care Med 2001;163(7):1626–31.
42. Beebe DW, Gozal D. Obstructive sleep apnea and the prefrontal cortex: towards a comprehensive model linking nocturnal upper airway obstruction to daytime cognitive and behavioral deficits. J Sleep Res 2002;11(1):1–16.
43. Kushida CA, Littner MR, Hirshkowitz M, et al. Practice parameters for the use of continous and bilevel positive airway pressure devices to treat adult patients with sleep-related breathing disorders. Sleep 2006;29(3):375–80.
44. Ancoli-Israel S, Palmer BW, Cooke JR, et al. Cognitive effects of treating obstructive sleep apnea in Alzheimer's disease: a randomized controlled study. J Am Geriatr Soc 2008;56(11):2076–81.
45. Chong MS, Avalon L, Marler M, et al. Continuous positive airway pressure reduces subjective daytime sleepiness in patients with mild to moderate Alzheimer's disease with sleep disordered breathing. J Am Geriatr Soc 2006; 54(5):777–81.

46. Cooke JR, Ayalon L, Palmer BW, et al. Sustained use of CPAP slows deterioration of cognition, sleep, and mood in patients with Alzheimer's disease and obstructive sleep apnea: a preliminary study. J Clin Sleep Med 2009;5(4):305–9.
47. Valencia-Flores M, Bliwise DL, Guilleminault C, et al. Cognitive function in patients with sleep apnea after acute nocturnal nasal continuous positive airway pressure (CPAP) treatment: sleepiness and hypoxemia effects. J Clin Exp Neuropsychol 1996;18(2):197–210.
48. Naegele B, Pepin JL, Levy P, et al. Cognitive executive dysfunction in patients with obstructive sleep apnea syndrome (OSAS) after CPAP treatment. Sleep 1998;21(4):392–7.
49. Macey PM, Henderson LA, Macey KE, et al. Brain morphology associated with obstructive sleep apnea. Am J Respir Crit Care Med 2002;166:1382–7.
50. Morrell MJ. Neural consequences of sleep-disordered breathing: the role of intermittent hypoxia. Adv Exp Med Biol 2006;588:75–88.
51. Tonon C, Vetrugno R, Lodi R, et al. Proton magnetic resonance spectroscopy study of brain metabolism in obstructive sleep apnea syndrome before and after continuous positive airway pressure treatment. Sleep 2007;30(3):305–11.
52. Macey PM, Kumar R, Woo MA, et al. Brain structure changes in obstructive sleep apnea. Sleep 2008;31(7):967–77.
53. Ficker JH, Feistel H, Moller C, et al. Changes in regional CNS perfusion in obstructive sleep apnea syndrome: initial SPECT studies with injected nocturnal 99m Tc-HMPAO. Pneumologie 1997;51(9):926–30.
54. Kumar R, Birrer BV, Macey PM, et al. Reduced mamillary body volume in patients with obstructive sleep apnea. Neurosci Lett 2008;438(3):330–4.
55. Shahar E, Whitney CW, Redline S, et al. Sleep-disordered breathing and cardiovascular disease: cross-sectional results of the sleep heart health study. Am J Respir Crit Care Med 2001;163(1):19–25.
56. Yaggi HK, Concato J, Kernan WN, et al. Obstructive sleep apnea as a risk factor for stroke and death. N Engl J Med 2005;353(19):2034–41.
57. Harbison J, Gibson GJ, Birchall D, et al. White matter disease and sleep-disordered breathing after acute stroke. Neurology 2003;61(7):959–63.
58. Wessendorf TE, Thilmann AF, Wang YM, et al. Fibrinogen levels and obstructive sleep apena in ischemic stroke. Am J Respir Crit Care Med 2000;162(6):2039–42.
59. Bokinsky G, Miller M, Ault K, et al. Spontaneous platelet activation and aggregation during obstructive sleep apnea and its response to therapy with nasal continuous positive airway pressure. A preliminary investigation. Chest 1995;108(3):625–30.
60. Lee SA, Amis TC, Byth K, et al. Heavy snoring as a cause of carotid artery atherosclerosis. Sleep 2008;31(9):1207–13.
61. Guardiola JJ, Matheson PJ, Clavijo LC, et al. Hypercoagulability in patients with obstructive sleep apnea. Sleep Med 2001;2(6):517–23.
62. Bliwise DL. Is sleep apnea a cause of reversible dementia in old age? J Am Geriatr Soc 1996;44(11):1408–9.
63. Redline S, Kirchner HL, Quan SF, et al. The effects of age, sex, ethnicity, and sleep-disordered breathing on sleep architecture. Arch Intern Med 2004;164(4):406–18.
64. Boselli M, Parrino L, Smerieri A, et al. Effect of age on EEG arousals in normal sleep. Sleep 1998;21(4):351–7.
65. Weitzman ED. Sleep and aging. In: Katzman R, Terry RD, editors. The neurology of aging. Philadelphia: Davis; 1983. p. 167–88.

66. Campbell N, Boustani M, Limbil T, et al. The cognitive impact of anticholinergics: a clinical review. Clin Interv Aging 2009;4(1):225–33.

67. Bowen JD, Larson EB. Drug-induced cognitive impairment. Defining the problem and finding solutions. Drugs Aging 1993;3(4):349–57.

68. Glass J, Lanctot KL, Herrmann N, et al. Sedative hypnotics in older people with insomnia: meta-analysis of risks and benefits. BMJ 2005;331(7526):1169.

69. Dolder C, Nelson M, McKinsey J. Use of non-benzodiazepine hypnotics in the elderly: are all agents the same? CNS Drugs 2007;21(5):389–405.

70. Dolan-Sewell RT, Riley WT, Hunt CE. NIH State-of-the-Science conference on chronic insomnia. J Clin Sleep Med 2005;1:335–6.

71. Bloom HG, Ahmed I, Alessi C, et al. Evidence-based recommendations for the assessment and management of sleep disorders in older persons. J Am Geriatr Soc 2009;57:761–89.

72. Johnson MW, Suess PE, Griffiths RR. Ramelteon: a novel hypnotic lacking abuse liability and sedative adverse effects. Arch Gen Psychiatry 2006;63:1149–57.

73. Zammit G, Wang-Weigand S, Rosenthal M, et al. Effect of ramelteon on middle-of-the-night balance in older adults with chronic insomnia. J Clin Sleep Med 2009; 5(1):34–40.

74. Minzenberg MJ, Carter CS. Modafinil: a review of neurochemical actions and effects on cognition. Neuropsychopharmacology 2008;33(7):1477–502.

75. Nishino S, Okuro M. Armodafinil for excessive daytime sleepiness. Drugs Today (Barc) 2008;44(6):395–414.

76. Peters KR, Ray L, Smith V, et al. Changes in the density of stage 2 sleep spindles following motor learning in young and older adults. J Sleep Res 2008;17(1): 23–33.

77. Stickgold R, Walker MP. Sleep-dependent memory consolidation and reconsolidation. Sleep Med 2007;8(4):331–43.

Endocrine Aspects of Healthy Brain Aging

Nazem Bassil, MD[a], John E. Morley, MB, BCh[b,c],*

KEYWORDS

• Hormones • Cognition • Metabolic alteration

The concept that hormones can alter behavior is not new; Aretaeus the Cappadocian stated that hypogonadism in men was related to altered (effeminate) behavior.[1–3] The original description of Graves disease (hyperthyroidism) in the nineteenth century included a description of associated anxiety. Myxedema madness associated with goiter was also recognized. Behavior changes have been reported in Addison and Cushing disease. Depression has commonly been considered a symptom of various endocrinopathies.

This review does not concentrate on these well-known psychiatric manifestations of endocrine diseases, but concentrates on the more subtle effects of hormones and metabolic alteration seen in many older persons. The article focuses predominately on the role of hormones in cognition, as dementia and mild cognitive impairment are major problems in the older individual.[4–8]

DIABETES MELLITUS AND INSULIN RESISTANCE

Studies[9–13] from various populations have consistently shown an association between diabetes and cognitive decline or dementia. Hyperglycemia leads to cognitive decline in animals and humans.[14–16] Diabetes is associated with a 50% to 100% increase in risk of Alzheimer disease (AD) and of dementia overall and a 100% to 150% increased risk of vascular dementia.[17] Higher postprandial plasma glucose levels were associated with greater declines in cognitive performance.[18] An inverse correlation has been noted between some cognitive measures and hemoglobin A1C levels, suggesting that worse glycemic control may be associated with greater cognitive decline.[19]

The relationship between diabetes and dementia of the Alzheimer type is not clear.[20] The mechanism by which diabetes may increase dementia risk is uncertain;

[a] Department of Neurology and Psychiatry, Division of Geriatric Psychiatry, Saint Louis University, St Louis, MO 63104, USA
[b] Department of Internal Medicine, Division of Geriatric Medicine, Saint Louis University School of Medicine, 1402 South Grand Boulevard, M238, St Louis, MO 63104, USA
[c] GRECC, VA Medical Center, St Louis, MO 63125, USA
* Corresponding author. Department of Internal Medicine, Division of Geriatric Medicine, Saint Louis University School of Medicine, 1402 South Grand Boulevard, M238, St Louis, MO 63104. *E-mail address:* morley@slu.edu (J.E. Morley).

Clin Geriatr Med 26 (2010) 57–74
doi:10.1016/j.cger.2009.12.004
0749-0690/10/$ – see front matter. Published by Elsevier Inc.

it does not seem to be mediated entirely through vascular disease.[21] There is a pivotal role for brain insulin resistance and insulin deficiency as mediators of cognitive impairment and neurodegeneration, particularly AD. Insulin and insulinlike growth factors (IGFs) regulate neuronal survival, energy metabolism, and plasticity, which are required for learning and memory.[22] The neurodegeneration associated with peripheral insulin resistance is likely effected via a liver-brain axis whereby toxic lipids, including ceramides, cross the blood-brain barrier and cause brain insulin resistance, oxidative stress, neuroinflammation, and cell death. Insulin resistance is present in most diabetic patients and is associated with compensatory hyperinsulinemia.[23,24]

The Honolulu-Asia Aging Study[25] demonstrated that the effect of high levels of insulin on the risk of dementia was independent of diabetes and blood glucose. Increased peripheral insulin levels are associated with reduced brain atrophy and cognitive impairment in patients with early AD, suggesting a role for insulin signaling in the pathophysiology of AD.[26] A relationship between insulin and amyloid-β protein metabolism is being studied. Insulin and amyloid-β protein are degraded by the insulin-degrading protein (**Fig. 1**). This degradation suggests that high insulin levels inhibit the degradation of amyloid-β protein. It has been reported that patients who are treated with insulin had the highest incidence of dementia.[27] Diabetes is also associated with an increased incidence of depression.[28] This depression can lead to poor compliance and cognitive dysfunction.[29] In addition, hypoglycemia is associated with delirium, and repeated hypoglycemia episodes are believed to produce permanent damage to the brain.[30,31]

HYPERLIPIDEMIA

Lipid metabolism is likely to be an important pathway in amyloid-β protein deposition, τ phosphorylation, and disruption of synaptic plasticity and neurodegenerative end points.[32,33] Hypercholesterolemia may increase the risk of dementia.[34,35] Epidemiologic studies have established an association in young-old individuals between cognitive decline or incident dementia, higher dietary intake of saturated fats, transunsaturated fats, or cholesterol,[36,37] and vascular dementia.[38–40] Not all studies have confirmed this association.[41–43] Some have shown a lower risk of dementia with

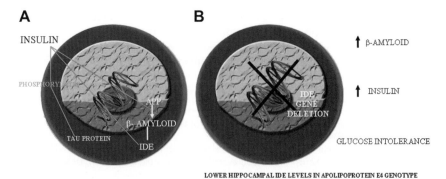

Fig. 1. (A) Insulin increases conversion of APP to amyloid-β protein, which at low levels enhances memory. At higher levels insulin is degraded by insulin-degrading enzyme (IDE), decreasing degradation of amyloid-β protein and raising it to pathologic levels at which it inhibits memory, causes oxidative damage, and forms insoluble plaques. (B) In IDE gene deletion animals there is an increase in amyloid-β protein and insulin. Persons with the apoE4 genotype have lower hippocampal levels of IDE.

high cholesterol levels in old age.[44] Some longitudinal studies indicate that, as with body mass index, serum cholesterol levels may decrease in the early stages of dementia, limiting the ability to see an effect of hypercholesterolemia on dementia risk when the measurements are made later in life.[45]

This finding has led to studies measuring the effect of cholesterol-lowering therapies (specifically the statin drugs) on the risk of dementia, which have shown mixed results. The treatment of hypercholesterolemia with statins impedes large-vessel atherosclerosis and its consequences. In addition, it may trigger various metabolic effects on the brain that may be related to AD pathogenesis.[46] Some epidemiologic studies[47] have shown a negative association between statin use and AD risk, and several mechanisms have been postulated.

Retrospective studies have suggested that statins may prevent the development of dementia.[48,49] This potential effect could be a direct association between amyloid processing and cholesterol in the brain,[50] or an indirect effect via decreasing the risk of stroke, because even small cerebral infarcts worsen the severity of AD.[51]

The efficacy of statins in reducing the incidence of dementia, the degree of age-related cognitive decline, or the neuropathologic burden of AD has been found in some studies,[52,53] but is not consistent.[54] Two large, randomized controlled trials[53,55] failed to show that use of 3-hydroxy-3-methylglutaryl-coenzyme A reductase inhibitors (statins) reduced the incidence of dementia. A Cochrane review[55] concluded that the evidence for a causal association was not yet present and there is no definitive evidence that treatment of hyperlipidemia leads to healthy brain aging.[56]

GROWTH HORMONE AND IGF-I

Growth hormone secretion declines approximately 14% per decade, and serum IGF-I levels decline in parallel.[57] There is a significant correlation between IGF-1 levels and cognition. IGF-1 level was significantly lower in patients with cognitive decline. A statistically nonsignificant but lower IGF-1 level was found in patients with pathologically wider radial width of the temporal horn (rWTH), which evaluates medial cerebral temporal lobe atrophy. A decrease in IGF-1 level related to a widening of the rWTH suggests an involvement of this hormone in hippocampus atrophy.[58]

LEPTIN

Leptin is a protein, secreted predominantly by adipocytes, which regulates appetite, energy balance, neuroendocrine function, and brain development.[59] Aging is associated with declining serum leptin levels, and with the development of leptin resistance.[60]

A growing body of research suggests that leptin may play a role in cognition. Leptin receptors and mRNA are widely expressed in the human brain and are involved in various processes across the central nervous system (CNS), including the hippocampus and neocortex.[61,62] Leptin play a role in hippocampal synaptic transmission and plasticity and is believed to underlie processes such as learning and memory.[63,64] A leptin deficiency may contribute to systemic and CNS abnormalities and aggravate insulin-controlled pathways, leading to disease progression.[65]

In animal models, leptin facilitates learning, spatial memory, and long-term potentiation.[66] Leptin modulates production and clearance of amyloid-β in rodent models.[67] Chronic administration of leptin resulted in a significant reduction in total brain amyloid-β load and an improvement in the cognitive performance of transgenic animal models.

Patients with AD have lower leptin levels than controls, inversely proportional to the severity of cognitive decline.[68] In addition, higher serum leptin in elderly individuals seems to protect against cognitive decline, independent of comorbidities and body fat.[69] These observations suggest that a leptin replacement therapy may be beneficial for patients with cognitive impairment.

METABOLIC SYNDROME

The metabolic syndrome is a cluster of cardiovascular risk factors, which include visceral obesity, hypertension, insulin resistance, hypertriglyceridemia, and low high-density lipoprotein cholesterol. Different components of the metabolic syndrome are associated with dementia. Untreated hypertension is associated with vascular dementia.[70] Hypertriglyceridemia can lead to delirium and cognitive impairment in animals and humans.[71] In 1 study,[72] the prevalence of AD was significantly higher in patients with metabolic syndrome. However, this association remains controversial. One case control study[73] found an association between the metabolic syndrome and AD. In a cohort study,[74] the metabolic syndrome was weakly associated with incident vascular dementia, but not AD. Other longitudinal studies of the metabolic syndrome and cognitive decline in older patients have found either no association or increased cognitive decline only in patients who also had increased markers of inflammation such as serum C-reactive protein and interleukin-6.[75]

TESTOSTERONE AND COGNITIVE FUNCTION

In men, testosterone levels decline at the rate of about 1% per year from 30 years of age.[76] Bioavailable testosterone levels (levels that are free or weakly bound to albumin) decline at almost twice that rate.[77] Between 30% and 60% of men in their 70s are hypogonadal.[78] Hypogonadism is strongly associated with a loss of muscle strength and frailty with aging.[79,80] The effects of hypogonadism on cognition are not so clear. Animal studies have shown that testosterone can improve memory, possibly by reducing amyloid-β peptide production.[81]

Testosterone plays an important role in brain functioning. Subclinical androgen deficiency was hypothesized to enhance the expression of amyloid-β–related peptides in vivo.[82] Age-related decreases in bioavailable testosterone predicted age-related decline in visual and verbal memory.[83] Men with a higher ratio of total testosterone to sex hormone binding globulin (SHBG) had a reduced incidence of AD[84] and patients with AD had a lower ratio of total testosterone to SHBG compared with age-matched controls.[85] In the Baltimore Longitudinal Study of Aging, a prospective longitudinal study risk for AD was reduced by 26% for each 10-unit (nmoL/nmoL) increase in free testosterone at 2, 5, and 10 years before AD diagnosis[86] Altered testosterone levels in AD may precede rather than follow diagnosis.[84] Low testosterone levels are also associated with mild cognitive impairment.[87]

There is evidence for a strong correlation between testosterone levels and cognitive performance such as spatial abilities or mathematical reasoning.[88] Recent animal experiments provide evidence that depletion of androgens results in increased pathologic conditions associated with AD, including increased antibody levels and hyperphosphorylated τ and increased neuronal death.[89] Testosterone and dihydro-testosterone have an effect on the upregulation of the hippocampal neurogenesis in adult male rodents.[90] In humans, higher bioavailable and free testosterone concentrations have each been associated with better performance in specific aspects of memory and cognitive function, with optimal processing capacity found in men between 35 and 90 years of age even after adjustment for potential confounders including age, educational attainment, and cardiovascular morbidity,[91,92] whereas total testosterone was not.[93] However, contradictory findings have also been reported. One cross-sectional study did not show a relationship between total or free testosterone and measures of working memory, speed/attention, or spatial relations in men aged from 48 to 80 years.[94] In another cross-sectional analysis of similarly aged men, no association was found between lower free testosterone levels and higher performance on spatial visualization tasks, and between higher free and total testosterone levels and poorer verbal memory and executive performance; however, there is a correlation with faster processing speed.[95] A possible source of conflicting results in these studies may stem from interactions between testosterone levels and other risk factors for cognitive impairment such as apolipoprotein E4 (apoE4) genotype[96] and systemic illness, which cause low testosterone.[87]

In men undergoing hormonal therapy for prostate cancer, suppression of endogenous testosterone synthesis and blockade of the androgen receptor resulted in a beneficial effect on verbal memory but an adverse effect on spatial ability.[97] They also had visuomotor slowing and slowed reaction times in several attentional domains.[98] Plasma amyloid levels increased as testosterone levels decreased. Discontinuation of treatment resulted in improved memory but not visuospatial abilities.[99] One of the possible protective mechanisms of action of testosterone would be through its conversion into estradiol (E_2), the most potent estrogen. Serum estradiol and testosterone levels were lower in men with AD compared with age-matched controls.[100,101] Estradiol may exert protective effects on the brain structures in aging patients.[102]

Trials of testosterone therapy in men to evaluate its effects on measures of cognitive function and memory to date have all been small and of a short duration and have shown mixed results.[85,103] Small-scale testosterone intervention trials in elderly men suggest that some cognitive deficits may be reversed, at least in part, by short-term testosterone supplementation.[104] Androgen supplementation in elderly hypogonadal men improves spatial cognition[105] and verbal fluency.[106] In elderly men without dementia, it may reduce working memory errors.[107] In addition, transdermal testosterone or dihydrotestosterone treatment in men aged 34 to 70 years improved verbal memory and spatial memory.[108] Intramuscular testosterone improved verbal and spatial memory and constructional abilities in nonhypogonadal men with mild cognitive impairment and early AD.[109] In this study of healthy men aged 50 to 90 years, intramuscular testosterone alone or in combination with anastrozole improved spatial memory, whereas verbal memory only improved in testosterone-treated men in the absence of anastrozole, raising the possibility that part of the effect of exogenous testosterone is mediated by its aromatization to estradiol.[109]

In men with AD, testosterone treatment appeared to improve quality of life without affecting measures of cognition.[110] In a randomized placebo-controlled crossover trial, intramuscular testosterone therapy resulted in decreased verbal memory.[111] Placebo-controlled randomized trials, one of which studied patients with Alzheimer dementia and low testosterone levels,[112] reported imprecise effects on several dimensions of cognition, none of which was significant after pooling.[113]

The associations of testosterone with depression are variable. Some, but not all, studies, have suggested a positive effect of testosterone replacement in persons with dysphoria.[114,115]

Therefore, there is some evidence that lower free testosterone seems to be associated with poorer outcomes on measures of cognitive function, particularly in older men, and testosterone therapy in hypogonadal men may have some benefit for cognitive performance and healthy brain aging. Larger, double-blind placebo-controlled trials that examine a wider range of cognitive tests account for genetic risk factor status and that are commenced early in the disease state are needed to examine the potential benefit of androgen supplementation as a possible therapy for AD.

ESTROGEN AND HORMONE THERAPY IN WOMEN

Estrogenic effects within the CNS and more specifically the hippocampus are mediated by estrogens receptors (ERs) α and β.[116,117] There is increasing laboratory evidence for a neuroprotective effect of estrogen that plays an important role in the modulation of neuroplasticity and behavior in the rodent and affects different brain regions involved in working memory, reference memory, and conditioned place preference.[90,118]

In women, unilateral and bilateral oophorectomies regardless of the indication preceding the onset of menopause are associated with an increased risk of cognitive impairment or dementia.[119] Several studies showed a significant reduction in risk of AD for women who used estrogen treatment after menopause.[120,121]

Estrogen may have a protective effect on the brain if given to women who underwent oophorectomy before menopause or if given in the perimenopausal and early postmenopausal years to women with natural menopause. By contrast, estrogen may have harmful effects on the brain if started many years after the onset of natural menopause. In addition, the data from the Women's Health Initiative (WHI) and the WHI Memory Study (WHIMS), a large randomized controlled trial of estrogen and progesterone replacement therapy in more than 7000 women 65 to 79 years of age, indicates that conjugated equine estrogen (CEE), initiated in the late postmenopausal period, does not improve global cognitive function and may adversely affect this outcome.[122–124] The effects on cognition were similar to those observed with CEE plus medroxyprogesterone acetate (MPA). Neither CEE nor CEE plus MPA should be initiated in older women for the purpose of protecting cognitive function and enhancing the brain during aging. Furthermore, at least 1 subgroup of women was at particularly high risk for the adverse effects of hormone therapy on cognition: women with low baseline cognitive function.[123]

These contradictory findings may be explained by an age-dependent effect of estrogen on the brain,[125,126] and there may be a critical age window for neuroprotection.[127] A large epidemiologic study indicated that estrogen exerts its protective effect only if taken during the onset of menopause and the first few years thereafter.[102,128]

DEHYDROEPIANDROSTERONE AND PREGNENOLONE

The adrenals secrete large amounts of dehydroepiandrosterone (DHEA) and DHEA sulfate (DHEAS) that are biotransformed into biologically active androgens and estrogens in peripheral tissues and in neuroactive steroids in the brain. There is a progressive, continuous decline of DHEAS levels with aging. In the longitudinal Baltimore study of healthy aging men, the decline in serum DHEAS levels was independent of cognitive status and cognitive decline. DHEA has been proposed to have many potential benefits in retarding diseases associated with aging, including cognitive impairment and dementia. Animal studies have shown a strong effect of DHEA on memory.[129–131] However, human studies do not support a benefit for DHEA on cognitive function.[132]

Pregnenolone is the precursor for all the steroids. As such, it is often considered the mother hormone. Our studies in mice found that low doses of pregnenolone increase learning and retention in mice.[133–135] These effects seem to involve interference with the inhibitory effect of γ butyric amino acid. Although some human studies have suggested that pregnenolone may increase attention, tests on learning and memory have been disappointing.

CORTISOL

Glucocorticoid hormones are important in the maintenance of many brain functions.[136] The glucocorticoid response to stressful stimuli is regulated by the hypothalamic-pituitary-adrenal (HPA) axis, which triggers the adrenal cortex to release glucocorticoids, which are crucial for many CNS functions,[137] including the prefrontal cortex (PFC),[138] a brain region critical for working memory, executive function, and extinction of learning.[139] Stress induced alterations of glutamatergic transmission in PFC, which is considered the core feature and fundamental pathologic condition of stress-related mental disorders with impaired working memory.[140,141]

Whereas chronic stress often produces detrimental effects on these measures, acute stress predominantly through the action of corticosteroid stress hormones within the context of a learning situation results in focused attention and improvements in memory.[142] Stress through glucocorticoids might have an inverted-U relationship to cognitive function, such that a moderate level has procognitive effects, whereas too low or too high levels are detrimental to cognitive processing.[143]

There is also a dysfunction in the HPA axis in AD, reflected by markedly increased basal levels of circulating cortisol[144] and a failure to show cortisol suppression after a dexamethasone challenge.[145] There is some evidence from animal studies to suggest an interaction between glucocorticoids and AD pathology, including amyloid precursor protein (APP) and τ accumulation.[146] The detrimental effects of cortisol seem to be directed at the hippocampus. The damaging effects of increased corticosteroid levels are mediated by the duration of exposure to corticosteroids or stress, the dose of corticosteroids and the vulnerability of the hippocampus, amygdala, and prefrontal cortex areas.[147,148] Patients with AD treated with prednisone exhibited impaired cognition compared with the placebo-treated cohort.[149]

Increased cortisol levels in the cerebrospinal fluid if patients with AD mirrored the presence of the apoE4 allele,[150] suggesting that apoE function was influencing circulating cortisol levels. There is a genetic link between glucocorticoid function and the risk for sporadic AD.[151]

VITAMIN D

Vitamin D is a steroid hormone that has long been known for its role in regulating body levels of calcium and phosphorus. Its biologic effects extend beyond control of mineral metabolism. Vitamin D levels have been shown to decline longitudinally with age.[152] The prevalence of vitamin D deficiency is common in elderly individuals, affecting up to 50% of older adults and a higher percentage of nursing-home residents.[153–155] Vitamin D deficiency occurs as a result of restricted sunlight exposure, reduced capacity of the skin to produce vitamin D, and reduced dietary intake.[156] Vitamin D has multiple biologic targets mediated by the vitamin D receptor (VDR), which is present on many cells including neurons.[157,158] The effects of vitamin D on the CNS have been described. In vitro studies and animal experiments suggest a role in the regulation of neurotransmission, the expression of neurotrophic factors, the stimulation of adult neurogenesis, calcium homeostasis, and detoxification.[159–161] Vitamin D may have a protective role in neurodegenerative diseases. Furthermore, there is a downregulation of VDRs in hippocampal cells in AD.[162]

There is no linear association between serum 25-hydroxyvitamin D (25[OH]D) and verbal memory performance in older adults.[163] Some studies showed that low

25(OH)D concentrations were associated with low cognitive status performance, whereas others did not.[163–167] Discrepancies may be explained, in part, by confounding variables such as age, education level, and level of physical activity.

Treatment with vitamin D for 8 and 12 months resulted in a higher density of neurons in the rat hippocampus.[168] In humans, following vitamin D supplementation, a modest increase in clock-drawing test performance, although not verbal fluency, was also observed over 4 weeks in 25 nursing-home residents with low 25(OH)D status at baseline.[169] Evidence from well-designed trials is lacking.

On the other hand, hypercalcemia, presumably caused by mild primary hyperparathyroidism, was a significant predictor for the development of cognitive decline.[170] There is an effect of serum intact parathyroid hormone (PTH) on cognitive performance[171,172] in patients with chronic renal failure and increased serum PTH levels, and there are various neurobehavioural abnormalities[173]; in elderly patients with primary hyperparathyroidism, dementia is frequently found and often alleviated after parathyroidectomy.[174]

GONADOTROPIN

The incidence of AD is higher in women than in men.[175] Neurofibrillary tangles and amyloid senile plaques are more substantial in women with AD, particularly women with APOE ε 4 compared with men with the disease.[176] The higher incidence of AD in women may possibly be caused by a rapid decline in the steroid hormone after menopause.[177] Luteinizing hormone (LH) is present in the brain and has the highest receptor levels in the hippocampus, a key processor of cognition that is severely deteriorated in AD. Plasma LH levels are increased in AD subjects.[178] Furthermore, increased levels of gonadotropins have also been found in individuals with Down syndrome, in whom dementia and Alzheimer-like symptoms usually develop with advancing age.[179]

High endogenous LH levels were associated with a lower cognitive score, especially in older women and in women who were depressed. Disproportionately well-preserved cognitive functioning was found for the oldest women who had high endogenous levels of follicle-stimulating hormone (FSH). The findings indicate that gonadotropins can affect cognitive functioning in older postmenopausal women, and that LH and FSH may exert contrasting effects.[180]

LH promotes the amyloidogenic processing of the amyloid-β precursor protein in vivo and in vitro, suggesting that LH may contribute to AD pathology through an amyloid-dependent mechanism. The increase of LH with the dysregulation of the hypothalamic-pituitary-gonadal axis at menopause and andropause is a physiologically relevant signal that could promote neurodegeneration in the aging brain.[181–183]

The regulation of the pituitary gonadotropins FSH and LH is under the control of complex feedback loops within the hypothalamic-pituitary-ovary axis that, in turn, regulate estrogen levels.[184] It remains to be determined if the changes in one or a combination of low levels of estrogen and high levels of gonadotropins associated with cognitive deficits in dementia can influence cognitive functioning for older postmenopausal women.

MELATONIN

Melatonin is capable of interfering with mitochondrial cell death pathways and activating survival pathways, both of which would be useful in treating AD. It is thought that reduced secretion of melatonin is associated with the development of neurodegenerative disease; blood concentrations of neurohormone melatonin are significantly decreased in patients with AD.[185]

The pineal gland enables spatiotemporal integration in cognitive processing. Melatonin could be a potential regulator in the processes that contribute to memory formation, long-term potentiation, and synaptic plasticity in the hippocampus and other brain regions. Melatonin has a role in mechanisms of consciousness, memory, and stress. There is an alteration under stressful conditions and in mental disorders.[186]

Melatonin has a role in AD and future therapeutic strategies could be directed at identifying and developing drugs from among the analogs of melatonin that may slow the progression of neurodegenerative diseases.

SUMMARY

There is a long history of hormones altering behavior and endocrinopathies playing a role in psychiatric disease. This review highlights the hormonal changes that occur with aging and the effects of these hormonal changes on the brain.

REFERENCES

1. Morley JE. A brief history of geriatrics. J Gerontol A Biol Sci Med Sci 2004;59: 1132–52.
2. Morley JE, Perry HM 3rd. Androgen deficiency in aging men: role of testosterone replacement therapy. J Lab Clin Med 2000;135:370–8.
3. Morley JE, Flood J, Silver AJ. Effects of peripheral hormones on memory and ingestive behaviors. Psychoneuroendocrinology 1992;17:391–9.
4. Lee M, Chodosh J. Dementia and life expectancy: what do we know? J Am Med Dir Assoc 2009;10:466–71.
5. Samus QM, Mayer L, Onyike CU, et al. Correlates of functional dependence among recently admitted assisted living residents with and without dementia. J Am Med Dir Assoc 2009;10:323–9.
6. Morley JE. Managing persons with dementia in the nursing home: high touch trumps high tech. J Am Med Dir Assoc 2008;9:139–46.
7. Kaufer DI, Williams CS, Braaten AJ, et al. Cognitive screening for dementia and mild cognitive impairment in assisted living: comparison of 3 tests. J Am Med Dir Assoc 2008;9:586–93.
8. Volicer L. Behaviors in advanced dementia. J Am Med Dir Assoc 2009;10:146.
9. Irie F, Fitzpatrick AL, Lopez OL, et al. Enhanced risk for Alzheimer disease in persons with type 2 diabetes and APOE {varepsilon}4: The Cardiovascular Health Study Cognition Study. Arch Neurol 2008;65(1):89–93.
10. Peila R, Rodriguez BL, Launer LJ. Type 2 diabetes, APOE gene, and the risk for dementia and related pathologies: the Honolulu-Asia Aging Study. Diabetes 2002;51(4):1256–62.
11. MacKnight C, Rockwood K, Awalt E, et al. Diabetes mellitus and the risk of dementia, Alzheimer's disease and vascular cognitive impairment in the Canadian Study of Health and Aging. Dement Geriatr Cogn Disord 2002;14(2):77–83.
12. Hassing LB, Johansson B, Nilsson SE, et al. Diabetes mellitus is a risk factor for vascular dementia, but not for Alzheimer's disease: a population-based study of the oldest old. Int Psychogeriatr 2002;14(3):239–48.
13. Schnaider Beeri M, Goldbourt U, Silverman JM, et al. Diabetes mellitus in midlife and the risk of dementia three decades later. Neurology 2004;63:1902–7.
14. Flood JF, Mooradian AD, Morley JE. Characteristics of learning and memory in steptozocin-induced diabetic mice. Diabetes 1999;39:1391–8.

15. Mooradian AD, Perryman K, Fitten J, et al. Cortical function in elderly non-insulin dependent diabetic patients. Behavioral and electrophysiologic studies. Arch Intern med 1988;148:2369–72.
16. Messinger-Rapport BJ, Thomas DR, Gammack JK, et al. Clinical update on nursing home medicine: 2008. J Am Med Dir Assoc 2008;9:460–75.
17. Biessels GJ, Staekenborg S, Brunner E, et al. Risk of dementia in diabetes mellitus: a systematic review. Lancet Neurol 2006;5(1):64–74 [Erratum in: Lancet Neurol 2006;5(2):113].
18. Abbatecola AM, Rizzo MR, Barbieri M, et al. Postprandial plasmaglucose excursions and cognitive functioning in aged type 2 diabetics. Neurology 2006;67(2): 235–40.
19. Munshi M, Grande L, Hayes M, et al. Cognitive dysfunction is associated with poor diabetes control in older adults. Diabetes Care 2006;29(8):1794–9.
20. Xu WL, Qiu CX, Wahlin A, et al. Diabetes mellitus and risk of dementia in the Kungsholmen project: a 6-year follow-up study. Neurology 2004;63(7):1181–6.
21. Biessels GJ, De Leeuw FE, Lindeboom J, et al. Increased cortical atrophy in patients with Alzheimer's disease and type 2 diabetes mellitus. J Neurol Neurosurg Psychiatr 2006;77(3):304–7.
22. Tong M, de la Monte SM. Ceramide-mediated neurodegeneration: relevance to diabetes-associated neurodegeneration. J Alzheimers Dis 2009;16: 705–14.
23. Steen E, Terry BM, Rivera EJ, et al. Impaired insulin and insulin-like growth factor expression and signaling mechanisms in Alzheimer's disease–is this type 3 diabetes? J Alzheimers Dis 2005;7:63–80.
24. Arboleda G, Huang TJ, Waters C, et al. Insulin-like growth factor-1-dependent maintenance of neuronal metabolism through the phosphatidylinositol 3-kinase-Akt pathway is inhibited by C2-ceramide in CAD cells. Eur J Neurosci 2007;25:3030–8.
25. Peila R, Rodriguez BL, White LR, et al. Fasting insulin and incident dementia in an elderly population of Japanese-American men. Neurology 2004;63(2): 228–33.
26. Burns JM, Donnelly JE, Anderson HS, et al. Peripheral insulin and brain structure in early Alzheimer disease. Neurology 2007;69(11):1094–104.
27. Ott A, Stolk RP, van Harskamp F, et al. Diabetes mellitus and the risk of dementia. The Rotterdam Study. Neurology 1999;53(9):1937–42.
28. Rosenthal MJ, Fajardo M, Gilmore S, et al. Hospitalization and mortality of diabetes in older adults. A 3-year prospective study. Diabetes Care 1998;21:231–5.
29. Mazza AD, Morley JE. Update on diabetes in the elderly and the application of current therapeutics. J Am Med Dir Assoc 2007;8:489–92.
30. Flaherty JH, Shay K, Weir C, et al. The development of a mental status vital sign for use across the spectrum of care. J Am Med Dir Assoc 2009;10:379–80.
31. Flaherty JH, Rudolph J, Shay K, et al. Delirium is a serious and under-recognized problem: why assessment of mental status should be the sixth vital sign. J Am Med Dir Assoc 2007;8:273–5.
32. Michikawa M. Cholesterol paradox: is high total or low HDL cholesterol level a risk for Alzheimer's disease? J Neurosci Res 2003;72(2):141–6.
33. Michikawa M. The role of cholesterol in pathogenesis of Alzheimer's disease: dual metabolic interaction between amyloid beta-protein and cholesterol. Mol Neurobiol 2003;27(1):1–12.
34. Whitmer RA, Sidney S, Selby J, et al. Midlife cardiovascular risk factors and risk of dementia in late life. Neurology 2005;64(2):277–81.

35. Solomon A, Kåreholt I, Ngandu T, et al. Serum cholesterol changes after midlife and late-life cognition: twenty-one-year follow-up study. Neurology 2007;68(10): 751–6.
36. Kalmijn S, van Boxtel MP, Ocké M, et al. Dietary intake of fatty acids and fish in relation to cognitive performance at middle age. Neurology 2004;62(2):275–80.
37. Engelhart MJ, Geerlings MI, Ruitenberg A, et al. Diet and risk of dementia. Does fat matter?: the Rotterdam Study. Neurology 2002;59(12):1915–21.
38. Moroney JT, Tang MX, Berglund L, et al. Low-density lipoprotein cholesterol and the risk of dementia with stroke. JAMA 1999;282(3):254–9.
39. Reitz C, Tang MX, Luchsinger J, et al. Relation of plasma lipids to Alzheimer disease and vascular dementia. Arch Neurol 2004;61(5):705–14.
40. Dufouil C, Richard F, Fievet N, et al. APOE genotype, cholesterol level, lipid-lowering treatment, and dementia: the Three-City Study. Neurology 2005; 64(9):1531–8.
41. Tan ZS, Seshadri S, Beiser A, et al. Plasma total cholesterol level as a risk factor for Alzheimer disease: the Framingham Study. Arch Intern Med 2003;163(9): 1053–7.
42. Reitz C, Luchsinger J, Tang MX, et al. Impact of plasma lipids and time on memory performance in healthy elderly without dementia. Neurology 2005; 64(8):1378–83.
43. Li G, Shofer JB, Kukull WA, et al. Serum cholesterol and risk of Alzheimer disease: a community-based cohort study. Neurology 2005;65(7):1045–50.
44. Mielke MM, Zandi PP, Sjögren M, et al. High total cholesterol levels in late life associated with a reduced risk of dementia. Neurology 2005;64(10):1689–95.
45. Stewart R, White LR, Xue QL, et al. Twenty-six-year change in total cholesterol levels and incident dementia: the Honolulu-Asia Aging Study. Arch Neurol 2007;64(1):103–7.
46. Kirsch C, Eckert GP, Mueller WE. Statin effects on cholesterol microdomains in brain plasma membranes. Biochem Pharmacol 2003;65(5):843–56.
47. Crisby M, Carlson LA, Winblad B. Statins in the prevention and treatment of Alzheimer disease. Alzheimer Dis Assoc Disord 2002;16(3):131–6.
48. Jick H, Zornberg GL, Jick SS, et al. Statins and the risk of dementia. Lancet 2000;356(9242):1627–31 [Erratum in: Lancet 2001;357(9255):562].
49. Rodriguez EG, Dodge HH, Birzescu MA, et al. Use of lipid-lowering drugs in older adults with and without dementia: a community-based epidemiological study. J Am Geriatr Soc 2002;50(11):1852–6.
50. Fassbender K, Simons M, Bergmann C, et al. Simvastatin strongly reduces levels of Alzheimer's disease beta -amyloid peptides Abeta 42 and Abeta 40 in vitro and in vivo. Proc Natl Acad Sci U S A 2001;98(10):5856–61.
51. Cramer C, Haan MN, Galea S, et al. Use of statins and incidence of dementia and cognitive impairment without dementia in a cohort study. Neurology 2008; 71(5):344–50.
52. Rea TD, Breitner JC, Psaty BM. Statin use and the risk of incident dementia: the Cardiovascular Health Study. Arch Neurol 2005;62(7):1047–51.
53. Heart Protection Study Collaborative Group. MRC/BHF Heart Protection Study of cholesterol lowering with simvastatin in 20,536 high-risk individuals: a randomised placebo-controlled trial. Lancet 2002;360(9326):7–22.
54. Bernick C, Katz R, Smith NL, et al. Statins and cognitive function in the elderly: the Cardiovascular Health Study. Neurology 2005;65(9):1388–94.
55. Scott HD, Laake K. Statins for the prevention of Alzheimer's disease. Cochrane Database Syst Rev 2001;(4):CD003160.

56. Essink-Bot ML, Pereria J, Packer C, et al. Cross-national comparability of burden of disease estimates: the European Disability Weights Project. Bull World Health Organ 2002;80(8):644–52.
57. Lamberts SWJ. The endocrinology of aging and the brain. Arch Neurol 2002;59: 1709–11.
58. Angelini A, Bendini C, Neviani F, et al. Insulin-like growth factor-1 (IGF-1): relation with cognitive functioning and neuroimaging marker of brain damage in a sample of hypertensive elderly subjects. Arch Gerontol Geriatr 2009;49(Suppl 1):5–12.
59. Harvey J. Leptin: a multifaceted hormone in the central nervous system. Mol Neurobiol 2003;28:245–58.
60. Isidori AM, Strollo F, Morè M, et al. Leptin and aging: correlation with endocrine changes in male and female healthy adult populations of different body weights. J Clin Endocrinol Metab 2000;85(5):1954–62.
61. Funahashi H, Yada T, Suzuki R, et al. Distribution, function, and properties of leptin receptors in the brain. Int Rev Cytol 2003;224:1–27.
62. O'Malley D, MacDonald N, Mizielinska S, et al. Leptin promotes rapid dynamic changes in hippocampal dendritic morphology. Mol Cell Neurosci 2007;35: 559–72.
63. Harvey J, Shanley LJ, O'Malley D, et al. Leptin: a potential cognitive enhancer? Biochem Soc Trans 2005;33:1029–32.
64. Irving AJ, Wallace L, Durakoglugil D, et al. Leptin enhances NR2B-mediated N-methyl-D-aspartate responses via a mitogen-activated protein kinase-dependent process in cerebellar granule cells. Neuroscience 2006;138:1137–48.
65. Tezapsidis N, Johnston JM, Smith MA, et al. Leptin: a novel therapeutic strategy for Alzheimer's disease. J Alzheimers Dis 2009;16(4):731–40.
66. Li XL, Aou S, Oomura Y, et al. Impairment of long-term potentiation and spatial memory in leptin receptor-deficient rodents. Neuroscience 2002;113(3):607–15.
67. Fewlass DC, Noboa K, Pi-Sunyer FX, et al. Obesity-related leptin regulates Alzheimer's Abeta. FASEB J 2004;18(15):1870–8.
68. Power DA, Noel J, Collins R, et al. Circulating leptin levels and weight loss in Alzheimer's disease patients. Dement Geriatr Cogn Disord 2001;12(2):167–70.
69. Holden KF, Lindquist K, Tylavsky FA, et al. Serum leptin level and cognition in the elderly: findings from the Health ABC Study. Neurobiol Aging 2009;30(9): 1483–9.
70. Joshi S, Morley JE. Cognitive impairment. Med Clin North Am 2006;90:769–87.
71. Farr SA, Yamada KA, Butterfield DA, et al. Obesity and hypertriglyceridemia produce cognitive impairment. Endocrinology 2008;149:2628–36.
72. Vanhanen M, Koivisto K, Moilanen L, et al. Association of metabolic syndrome with Alzheimer disease: a population-based study. Neurology 2006;67(5):843–7.
73. Razay G, Vreugdenhil A, Wilcock G. The metabolic syndrome and Alzheimer disease. Arch Neurol 2007;64(1):93–6.
74. Kalmijn S, Foley D, White L, et al. Metabolic cardiovascular syndrome and risk of dementia in Japanese-American elderly men. The Honolulu-Asia aging study. Arterioscler Thromb Vasc Biol 2000;20(10):2255–60.
75. Yaffe K, Kanaya A, Lindquist K, et al. The metabolic syndrome, inflammation, and risk of cognitive decline. JAMA 2004;292(18):2237–42.
76. Morley JE, Kaiser FE, Perry HM 3rd, et al. Longitudinal changes in testosterone, luteinizing hormone, and follicle-stimulating hormone in healthy older men. Metabolism 1997;46:410–3.
77. Morley JE, Patrick P, Perry HM 3rd. Evaluation of assays available to measure free testosterone. Metabolism 2002;51:554–9.

78. Wang C, Nieschlag E, Swerdloff RS, et al. ISA, ISSAM, EAU, EAA and ASA recommendations: investigation, treatment and monitoring of late-onset hypogonadism in males. Aging Male 2009;12:5–12.
79. Wittert GA, Chapman IM, Haren MT, et al. Oral testosterone undecanoate on visuospatial cognition, mood and quality of life in elderly men with low-normal gonadal status. Maturitas 2005;50:124–33.
80. Abelland van Kan G, Rolland YM, Morley JE, et al. Frailty: toward a clinical definition. J Am Med Dir Assoc 2008;9:71–2.
81. Flood JF, Farr SA, Kaiser FE, et al. Age-related decrease of plasma testosterone in SAMP8 mice: replacement improves age-related impairment of learning and memory. Physiol Behav 1995;57:669–73.
82. Gillett MJ, Martins RN, Clarnette RM, et al. Relationship between testosterone, sex hormone binding globulin and plasma amyloid beta peptide 40 in older men with subjective memory loss or dementia. J Alzheimers Dis 2003;5:267–9.
83. Morley JE, Kaiser F, Raum WJ, et al. Potentially predictive and manipulable blood serum correlates of aging in the healthy human male: progressive decreases in bioavailable testosterone, dehydroepiandrosterone sulfate, and the ratio of insulin-like growth factor 1 to growth hormone. Proc Natl Acad Sci U S A 1997;94:7537–42.
84. Moffat SD, Zonderman AB, Metter EJ, et al. Free testosterone and risk for Alzheimer disease in older men. Neurology 2004;62:188–93.
85. Hogervorst E, Bandelow S, Combrinck M, et al. Low free testosterone is an independent risk factor for Alzheimer's disease. Exp Gerontol 2004;39:1633–9.
86. Moffat SD. Effects of testosterone on cognitive and brain aging in elderly men. Ann N Y Acad Sci 2005;1055:80–92.
87. Chu LW, Tam S, Lee PW, et al. Bioavailable testosterone is associated with a reduced risk of amnestic mild cognitive impairment in older men. Clin Endocrinol (Oxf) 2008;68(4):589–98.
88. McKeever WF, Deyo A. Testosterone, dihydrotestosterone and spatial task performance of males. Bull Psychon Soc 1990;28:305–8.
89. Drummond ES, Harvey AR, Martins RN, et al. Androgens and Alzheimer's disease. Curr Opin Endocrinol Diabetes Obes 2009;16:254–9.
90. Galea LA, Uban KA, Epp JR, et al. Endocrine regulation of cognition and neuroplasticity: our pursuit to unveil the complex interaction between hormones, the brain, and behavior. Can J Exp Psychol 2008;62:247–60.
91. Yaffe K, Lui L-Y, Zmuda J, et al. Sex hormones and cognitive function in older men. J Am Geriatr Soc 2002;50:707–12.
92. Thilers PP, MacDonald SWS, Herlitz A. The association between endogenous free testosterone and cognitive performance: a population based study in 35 to 90 year-old men and women. Psychoneuroendocrinology 2006;31:565–76.
93. Yeap BB, Almeida OP, Hyde Z, et al. Higher serum free testosterone is associated with better cognitive function in older men, whilst total testosterone is not. The Health In Men Study. Clin Endocrinol 2008;68:404–12.
94. Yonker JE, Eriksson E, Nilsson L-G, et al. Negative association of testosterone on spatial visualisation in 35 to 80 year old men. Cortex 2006;42:376–86.
95. Martin DM, Wittert G, Burns NR, et al. Testosterone and cognitive function in ageing men: data from the Florey Adelaide Male Ageing Study (FAMAS). Maturitas 2007;57:182–94.
96. Burkhardt MS, Foster JK, Clarnet te RM, et al. Interaction between testosterone and apolipoprotein E e4 status on cognition in healthy older men. J Clin Endocrinol Metab 2006;91:1168–72.

97. Cherrier MM, Rose AL, Higano C. The effects of combined androgen blockade on cognitive function during the first cycle of intermittent androgen suppression in patients with prostate cancer. J Urol 2003;170:1808–11.

98. Salminen EK, Portin RI, Koskinen A, et al. Associations between serum testosterone fall and cognitive function in prostate cancer patients. Clin Cancer Res 2004;10:7575–82.

99. Almeida OP, Waterreus A, Spry N, et al. One year follow-up study of the association between chemical castration, sex hormones, beta-amyloid, memory and depression in men. Psychoneuroendocrinology 2004;29(8):1071–81.

100. Hogervorst E, Williams J, Budge M, et al. Serum total testosterone is lower in men with Alzheimer's disease. Neuro Endocrinol Lett 2001;22(3):163–8.

101. Bowen RL, Isley JP, Atkinson RL. An association of elevated serum gonadotropin concentrations and Alzheimer disease? J Neuroendocrinol 2000;12(4):351–4.

102. Gibbs RB, Gabor R. Estrogen and cognition: applying preclinical findings to clinical perspectives. J Neurosci Res 2003;74(5):637–43.

103. Beauchet O. Testosterone and cognitive function: current clinical evidence of a relationship. Eur J Endocrinol 2006;155:773–81.

104. Lyngdorf P, Hemmingsen L. Epidemiology of erectile dysfunction and its risk factors: a practice-based study in Denmark. Int J Impot Res 2004;16:105–11.

105. Orwoll ES, Oviatt SK, Biddle J, et al. Transdermal testosterone supplementation in normal older men. Proceedings of the 74th Meeting of The Endocrine Society, San Antonio, TX; 1992. p. 319.

106. Alexander GM, Swerdloff RS, Wang C, et al. Androgen-behavior correlations in hypogonadal men and eugonadal men. Horm Behav 1998;33:85–94.

107. Janowsky JS, Chavez B, Orwoll E. Sex steroids modify working memory. J Cogn Neurosci 2000;12:407–14.

108. Cherrier MM, Craft S, Matsumoto AH. Cognitive changes associated with supplementation of testosterone or dihydrotestosterone in mildly hypogonadal men: a preliminary report. J Androl 2003;24:568–76.

109. Cherrier MM, Matsumoto AM, Amory JK, et al. Testosterone improves spatial memory in men with Alzheimer disease and mild cognitive impairment. Neurology 2005;64:2063–8.

110. Lu PH, Masterman DA, Mulnard R, et al. Effects of testosterone on cognition and mood in male patients with mild Alzheimer disease and healthy elderly men. Arch Neurol 2006;63:177–85.

111. Maki PM, Ernst M, London ED, et al. Intramuscular testosterone treatment in elderly men: evidence of memory decline and altered brain function. J Clin Endocrinol Metab 2007;92:4107–14.

112. Tan RS, Culberson JW. An integrative review on current evidence of testosterone replacement therapy for the andropause. Maturitas 2003;45:15–27.

113. Kenny AM, Fabregas G, Song C, et al. Effects of testosterone on behavior, depression, and cognitive function in older men with mild cognitive loss. J Gerontol A Biol Sci Med Sci 2004;59:75–8.

114. Sih R, Morley JE, Kaiser FE, et al. Testosterone replacement in older hypogonadal men: a 12-month randomized controlled trial. J Clin Endocrinol Metab 1997;82:1661–7.

115. Zarrouf FA, Artz S, Griffith J, et al. Testosterone and depression: systematic review and meta-analysis. J Psychiatr Pract 2009;15:289–305.

116. Vasudevan N, Pfaff DW. Membrane-initiated actions of estrogens in neuroendocrinology: emerging principles. Endocr Rev 2007;28:1–19.

117. Levin ER. Integration of the extranuclear and nuclear actions of estrogen. Mol Endocrinol 2005;19:1951–9.
118. Moult PR, Harvey J. Hormonal regulation of hippocampal dendritic morphology and synaptic plasticity. Cell Adh Migr 2008;2:269–75.
119. Rocca WA, Bower JH, Maraganore DM, et al. Increased risk of cognitive impairment or dementia in women who underwent oophorectomy before menopause. Neurology 2007;69(11):1074–83.
120. LeBlanc ES, Janowsky J, Chan BK, et al. Hormone replacement therapy and cognition: systematic review and meta-analysis. JAMA 2001;285:1489–99.
121. Hogervorst E, Williams J, Budge M, et al. The nature of the effect of female gonadal hormone replacement therapy on cognitive function in postmenopausal women: a meta-analysis. Neuroscience 2000;101:485–512.
122. Shumaker SA, Legault C, Rapp SR, et al. Estrogen plus progestin and the incidence of dementia and mild cognitive impairment in postmenopausal women: the Women's Health Initiative Memory Study: a randomized controlled trial. JAMA 2003;289:2651–62.
123. Espeland MA, Rapp SR, Shumaker SA, et al. Conjugated equine estrogens and global cognitive function in postmenopausal women: Women's Health Initiative Memory Study. JAMA 2004;291(24):2959–68.
124. Shumaker SA, Legault C, Kuller L, et al. Conjugated equine estrogens and incidence of probable dementia and mild cognitive impairment in postmenopausal women: Women's Health Initiative Memory Study. JAMA 2004;291:2947–58.
125. Henderson VW, Benke KS, Green RC, et al. Postmenopausal hormone therapy and Alzheimer's disease risk: interaction with age. J Neurol Neurosurg Psychiatr 2005;76:103–5.
126. Siegfried T. Neuroscience: it's all in the timing. Nature 2007;445:359–61.
127. Gibbs RG. Long-term treatment with estrogen and progesterone enhances acquisition of a spatial memory task by ovariectomized aged rats. Neurobiol Aging 2000;21:107–16.
128. Zandi PP, Carlson MC, Plassman BL, et al. Hormone replacement therapy and incidence of Alzheimer disease in older women: the Cache County Study. JAMA 2002;288:2123–9.
129. Farr SA, Banks WA, Uezu K, et al. DHEAS improves learning and memory in aged SAMP8 mice but not in diabetic mice. Life Sci 2004;75:2775–85.
130. Haren MT, Malmstrom TK, Banks WA, et al. Lower serum DHEAS levels are associated with a higher degree of physical disability and depressive symptoms in middle-aged to older African American women. Maturitas 2007;57:347–60.
131. Morley JE. Hormones and the aging process. J Am geriatr Soc 2003;51 (Suppl 7):S333–7.
132. Grimley Evans J, Malouf R, Huppert F. Dehydroepiandrosterone (DHEA) supplementation for cognitive function in healthy elderly people. Cochrane Database Syst Rev 2006;(4):CD006221.
133. Flood JF, Farr SA, Johnson DA, et al. Peripheral steroid sulfatase inhibition potentiates improvement of memory retention for hippocampally administered dehydroepiandrosterone sulfate but not pregnenolone sulfate. Psychoneuroendocrinology 1999;24:799–811.
134. Flood JF, Morley JE, Roberts E. Pregnenolone sulfate enhances post-training memory processes when injected in very low doses into limbic system structures: the amygdale is by far the most sensitive. Proc Natl Acad Sci U S A 1995;92:10806–10.

135. Flood JF, Morley JE, Roberts E. Memory-enhancing effects in male mice of pregnenolone and steroids metabolically derived from it. Proc Natl Acad Sci U S A 1992;89:1567–71.

136. Lupien SJ, Wilkinson CW, Briere S, et al. The modulatory effects of corticosteroids on cognition: studies in young human populations. Psychoneuroendocrinology 2002;27:401–16.

137. Roozendaal. 1999 Curt P. Richter award. Glucocorticoids and the regulation of memory consolidation. Psychoneuroendocrinology 2000;25(3): 213–38.

138. McEwen BS. Physiology and neurobiology of stress and adaptation: central role of the brain. Physiol Rev 2007;87:873–904.

139. Stuss DT, Knight RT, editors. Principles of frontal lobe function. New York: Oxford University Press; 2002. p. 90–107.

140. Yuen EY, Liu W, Karatsoreos IN, et al. Acute stress enhances glutamatergic transmission in prefrontal cortex and facilitates working memory. Proc Natl Acad Sci U S A 2009;106:14075–9.

141. Mizoguchi K, Ishige A, Takeda S, et al. Endogenous glucocorticoids are essential for maintaining prefrontal cortical cognitive function. J Neurosci 2004;24: 5492–9.

142. Joels M, Pu Z, Wiegert O, et al. Learning under stress: How does it work? Trends Cogn Sci 2006;10:152–8.

143. Joels M. Corticosteroid effects in the brain: U-shape it. Trends Pharmacol Sci 2006;27:244–50.

144. Swanwick GR, Kirby M, Bruce I, et al. Hypothalamic-pituitary-adrenal axis dysfunction in Alzheimer's disease: lack of association between longitudinal and cross-sectional findings. Am J Psychiatry 1998;155(2):286–9.

145. Näsman B, Olsson T, Seckl JR, et al. Abnormalities in adrenal androgens, but not of glucocorticoids, in early Alzheimer's disease. Psychoneuroendocrinology 1995;20(1):83–94.

146. Green KN, Billings LM, Roozendaal B, et al. Glucocorticoids increase amyloid-beta and tau pathology in a mouse model of Alzheimer's disease. J Neurosci 2006;26:9047–56.

147. Tsolaki M, Kounti F, Karamavrou S, et al. Severe psychological stress in elderly individuals: a proposed model of neurodegeneration and its implications. Am J Alzheimers Dis Other Demen 2009;24(2):85–94.

148. Lee BK, Glass TA, McAtee MJ, et al. Association of salivary cortisol with cognitive function in the Baltimore memory study. Arch Gen Psychiatry 2007;64:810–8.

149. Aisen PS. Anti-inflammatory therapy for Alzheimer's disease: implications of the prednisone trial. Acta Neurol Scand, Suppl 2000;176:85–9.

150. Peskind ER, Wilkinson CW, Petrie EC, et al. Increased CSF cortisol in AD is a function of APOE genotype. Neurology 2001;56(8):1094–8.

151. de Quervain DJ, Poirier R, Wollmer MA, et al. Glucocorticoid-related genetic susceptibility for Alzheimer's disease. Hum Mol Genet 2004;13(1):47–52.

152. Perry HM 3rd, Horowitz M, Morley JE, et al. Longitudinal changes in serum 25-hydroxyvitamin D in older people. Metabolism 1999;48:1028–32.

153. Gloth FM, Gundberg CM, Hollis BW, et al. Vitamin D deficiency in homebound elderly persons. JAMA 1995;274:1683–6.

154. Morley JE. Should all long-term care residents receive vitamin D? J Am Med Dir Assoc 2007;8:69–70.

155. Drinka PJ, Krause PF, Nest LJ, et al. Determinants of vitamin D levels in nursing home residents. J Am Med Dir Assoc 2007;8:76–9.

156. van der Wielen RP, Lowik MR, van den Berg H, et al. Serum vitamin D concentrations among elderly people in Europe. Lancet 1995;346:207–10.
157. Kalueff AV, Tuohimaa P. Neurosteroid hormone vitamin D and its utility in clinical nutrition. Curr Opin Clin Nutr Metab Care 2007;10:12–9.
158. Buell JS, Dawson-Hugues B. Vitamin D and neurocognitive dysfunction: preventing "D"ecline? Mol Aspects Med 2008;29:415–22.
159. McCann JC, Ames BN. Is there convincing biological or behavioral evidence linking vitamin D deficiency to brain dysfunction? FASEB J 2008;22: 982–1001.
160. Garcion E, Wion-Barbot N, Montero-Menei CN, et al. New clues about vitamin D functions in the nervous system. Trends Endocrinol Metab 2002;13:100–5.
161. Bourre JM. Effects of nutrients (in food) on the structure and function of the nervous system: update on dietary requirements for brain. Part 1: micronutrients. J Nutr Health Aging 2006;10:377–85.
162. Brewer LD, Thibault V, Chen KC, et al. Vitamin D hormone confers neuroprotection in parallel with downregulation of L-type calcium channel expression in hippocampal neurons. J Neurosci 2001;21:98–108.
163. McGrath J, Scragg R, Chant D, et al. No association between serum 25-hydroxyvitamin D3 level and performance on psychometric tests in NHANES III. Neuroepidemiology 2007;29:49–54.
164. Jorde R, Waterloo K, Saleh F, et al. Neuropsychological function in relation to serum parathyroid hormone and serum 25-hydroxyvitamin D levels: the Tromsø study. J Neurol 2006;253:464–70.
165. Wilkins CH, Sheline YI, Roe CM, et al. Vitamin D deficiency is associated with low mood and worse cognitive performance in older adults. Am J Geriatr Psychiatry 2006;14:1032–340.
166. Przybelski RJ, Binkley NC. Is vitamin D important for preserving cognition? A positive correlation of serum 25-hydroxyvitamin D concentration with cognitive function. Arch Biochem Biophys 2007;460:202–5.
167. Oudshoorn C, Mattace-Raso FU, Van Der Velde N, et al. Higher serum vitamin D3 levels are associated with better cognitive test performance in patients with Alzheimer's disease. Dement Geriatr Cogn Disord 2008;25:539–43.
168. Landfield PW, Cadwallader-Neal L. Long-term treatment with Calcitriol (1,25 (OH) 2 vit D3) retards a biomarker of hippocampal aging in rates. Neurobiol Aging 1998;19:469–77.
169. Przybelski R, Agrawal S, Krueger D, et al. Rapid correction of low vitamin D status in nursing home residents. Osteoporos Int 2008;19:1621–8.
170. Tilvis RS, Kähönen-Väre MH, Jolkkonen J, et al. Predictors of cognitive decline and mortality of aged people over a 10-year period. J Gerontol 2004;59:268–74.
171. Schram MT, Trompet S, Kamper AM, et al. Serum calcium and cognitive function in old age. J Am Geriatr Soc 2007;55:1786–92.
172. Khachaturian ZS. Calcium hypothesis of Alzheimer's disease and brain aging. Ann N Y Acad Sci 1994;747:1–11.
173. Smogorzewski MJ. Central nervous dysfunction in uremia. Am J Kidney Dis 2001;38(Suppl 1):S122–8.
174. Ohrvall U, Akerstrom G, Ljunghall S, et al. Surgery for sporadic primary hyperparathyroidism in the elderly. World J Surg 1994;18:612–8.
175. Farrer LA, Cupples LA, Myers RH, et al. Effects of age, sex, and ethnicity on the association between apolipoprotein E genotype and Alzheimer disease: a meta-analysis. APOE and Alzheimer Disease Meta Analysis Consortium. JAMA 1997; 278:1349–56.

176. Corder E, Ghebremedhin E, Taylor M, et al. The biphasic relationship between regional brain senile plaque and neurofibrillary tangle distributions: modification by age, sex and APOE polymorphism. Ann N Y Acad Sci 2004;1019:24–8.

177. Burkhardt M, Foster J, Clarnette R, et al. Estrogen replacement therapy may improve memory functioning in the absence of APOE ε4. J Alzheimers Dis 2004;6:221–8.

178. Bowen R, Smith M, Harris P, et al. Elevated luteinizing hormone expression co-localizes with neurons vulnerable to Alzheimer's disease pathology. J Neurosci Res 2002;70:514–8.

179. Bowen R, Verdile G, Liu T, et al. Luteinizing hormone, a reproductive regulator that modulates the processing of the amyloid-beta precursor protein and amyloid-beta deposition. J Biol Chem 2004;279:20539–45.

180. Rodrigues MA, Verdile G, Foster JK, et al. Gonadotropins and cognition in older women. J Alzheimers Dis 2008;13:267–74.

181. Meethal SV, Smith MA, Bowen RL, et al. The gonadotropin connection in Alzheimer's disease. Endocrine 2005;26:317–26.

182. Webber KM, et al. The contribution of luteinizing hormone to Alzheimer disease pathogenesis. Clin Med Res 2007;5:177–83.

183. Short R, Bowen R, O'Brien P, et al. Elevated gonadotropin levels in patients with Alzheimer disease. Mayo Clin Proc 2001;76:906–9.

184. Manly J, Merchant C, Jacobs D, et al. Endogenous estrogen levels and Alzheimer's disease among postmenopausal women. Neurology 2000;54: 833–7.

185. Wang X. The antiapoptotic activity of melatonin in neurodegenerative diseases. C J Pineal Res 2008;44(4):341–7.

186. Bob P, Fedor-Freybergh P. Melatonin, consciousness and traumatic stress. Melatonin, consciousness, and traumatic stress. J Pineal Res 2008;44:341–7.

Healthy Brain Aging: Role of Exercise and Physical Activity

Yves Rolland, MD, PhD[a,b,c,d,*], Gabor Abellan van Kan, MD[c,d],
Bruno Vellas, MD, PhD[a,b,c,d]

KEYWORDS

- Exercise • Cognition • Dementia • Physical activity
- Prevention

During the last 2 decades, it has been shown that the risk of numerous chronic diseases, such as congestive heart disease[1] or colon[2] and breast[3] cancer, can be reduced by increasing physical activity. The benefits that exercise can provide to brain functioning have been less thoroughly studied. However, the occurrence of dementia can be attributed to an accumulation of risk and protective factors during the lifespan,[4] and physical activity may contribute to the maintenance of a healthy aging brain. Recently, arguments from epidemiologic and basic research have emphasized that inactivity, a modifiable lifestyle factor, may affect age-related cognitive decline and the development of Alzheimer disease (AD).

Clinical and basic research in this area has intensified. Evidence suggests that potential preventive strategies such as a physically active lifestyle may help to delay the onset of cognitive decline and slow down disease progression. Such a nonpharmacologic therapeutic approach may be an appealing low-cost, low-risk alternative treatment of this major public health priority. In 2007, there were more than 5 million people in the United States with AD and there is still no pharmacologic treatment. Even a modest decrease in the incidence of the disease would have a significant effect on social and economic cost. It has been reported that a 5-year delay in the onset of dementia would result in a 50% decrease in the number of dementia cases.[5] In the absence of curative treatment, physical exercise seems a reasonable basis for prevention trials.[6] Only a few large randomized controlled trials (RCTs)[7,8] have been

Financial disclosure statement: Yves Rolland, Gabor Abellan, and Bruno Vellas have reported no financial or other conflicts of interest that might bias their work.

[a] Inserm U558, Avenue J. Guesdes, F-31073 Toulouse, France
[b] University of Toulouse III, F-31073 Toulouse, France
[c] Department of Geriatric Medicine, CHU Toulouse, Avenue de Casselardit, F-31059 Toulouse, France
[d] Service de Médecine Interne et de Gérontologie Clinique, Pavillon Junod, 170 avenue de Casselardit, Hôpital La Grave-Casselardit, 31300 Toulouse, France
* Corresponding author. Service de Médecine Interne et de Gérontologie Clinique, Pavillon Junod, 170 avenue de Casselardit, Hôpital La Grave-Casselardit, 31300 Toulouse, France.
E-mail address: rolland.y@chu-toulouse.fr (Y. Rolland).

conducted to show the benefit of physical activity on brain health. They support the benefit of physical activity on cognitive decline but none have shown that physical activity can prevent dementia. Trials involving physical activity in the prevention of cognitive decline and dementia have specific design challenges. Subjects who agree to engage in physical activity programs are likely to differ in many other lifestyle domains.[6] It is difficult to maintain compliance with a physical activity program for a long period, and it is difficult to assess the program. Like other nonpharmacologic trials, clinical research on physical activity is characterized by the impossibility of maintaining double-blind conditions, and the difficulty of defining an adequate control group. Despite these difficulties, the results of a well-designed RCT are needed.

In addition to many other reasons for engaging in physical activity, preserving brain health could be a strong and convincing argument for promoting activity in the population and could have a major effect on medical practice and public health education.

At present, there are no specific recommendations for physical programs to prevent cognitive decline, mainly because of the lack of RCTs. However, the strategy to prevent AD may target multiple aspects of lifestyle habits, including specific physical activity programs.

PHYSICAL ACTIVITY AND THE PREVENTION OF DEMENTIA, AD, OR COGNITIVE DECLINE
Clinical Research

All clinical evidence related to the prevention of dementia or AD by physical activity is derived from case-control studies and cross-sectional and longitudinal epidemiologic studies. There is currently no evidence, based on RCTs, to state that physical activity is effective in preventing or delaying the onset of dementia or AD. In a recent review,[9] 24 longitudinal epidemiologic studies were reported evaluating the possible effect of physical activity on cognitive decline, dementia, or AD. Most of them found an association between physical activity and cognitive decline or dementia, suggesting a protective effect of physical activity. Recently, 2 RCTs reported an improvement of cognitive function in an elderly population.[7,8]

Most of the current clinical evidence for the benefits of physical activity on the prevention of AD relies on epidemiologic studies.[9] Most of these studies investigated the relationship between physical activity and the risk of dementia or AD in particular. Others examined the relationship between physical activity and risk of cognitive decline. Despite similar outcomes, these longitudinal epidemiologic studies differ in many respects. However, the prospective cohort studies that have assessed the protective role of regular physical activity highlighted a significant and independent preventive effect of physical activity on cognitive decline or dementia. Most of the longitudinal epidemiologic studies that evaluated the association between physical activity and dementia or cognitive decline are reported in **Tables 1** and **2**. All these results were controlled for potential confounders underlying dementia and diminished physical activity. Five of the 16 longitudinal epidemiologic studies failed to find a statistically significant association between physical activity and dementia, and 2 of the 16 failed for cognitive decline (see **Table 2**).

Definitive conclusions based on these observational results must be discussed carefully as these epidemiologic studies are exposed to many sources of bias. In most of the studies the reliability of the physical activity assessment is questionable. The assessment of physical activity relies on 1 single question, a composite score based on physical activity during leisure and at work, and estimated average energy expenditure. Few research protocols have used validated standardized physical activity scales. The collection of self-reported activities also introduces a reporting bias. The type, frequency, and duration of activity are usually not quantified. Physical activity is assessed at study baseline but this assessment may not correspond to a mean stable and long-term regular activity and even less to activity over the subject's lifetime. The time elapsing between physical activity assessment and the onset of dementia or cognitive decline is variable. The mean follow-up between physical activity assessment and cognitive assessment varies from 2.5 to 21 years. An important limitation of these epidemiologic studies is that initial cognitive decline is associated with functional decline.[33–35] Inactivity may be a manifestation of the early phase of dementia rather than a risk factor. Most epidemiologic studies have tried to reduce this potential effect of behavior changes on physical activity in the early phase of AD by excluding subjects with low cognitive function at baseline or those who converted to AD in the early phases of follow-up. However, behavior disturbances such as depression, not assessed at baseline, usually precede AD and result in low physical activity.[36] The mean follow-up is short (3–7 years) compared with the decade or more before pathologic changes begin to be symptomatic and enable the diagnosis of dementia to be confirmed. Only 1 study investigated the long-term association between midlife physical activity and the risk of dementia or AD.[23] Another limitation in interpreting these epidemiologic studies is that despite adjustment for several potential confounders, sedentary participants differ from exercisers in many ways. Numerous other potential confounders may influence the relationship between exercise and risk of dementia. Physical activity involves cognitive functions (in addition to energy expenditure and mobility) that may enhance cognitive performances. Physical, social, and cognitive activities usually overlap. It is thus difficult to ascertain the specific and individual effect of each component on brain functioning.

Case-control studies also suggest that physical activities may have a direct influence on the neuropathology of AD. Most of these studies found that elderly participants who performed better on cognitive testing self-reported higher levels of physical activities in their past.[37,38] Physically fit aged individuals performed better in cognitive tests exploring reasoning, working memory, vocabulary, and reaction time than their sedentary counterparts. For example, in 1990, Broe and colleagues[39] reported that a low level of physical activity in the recent and the distant past was associated with AD. Others have reported that patients with AD were less active during their adulthood than subjects without dementia.[40–45] These case-control studies are even more prone to methodological bias.

The beneficial effects of physical exercise on the cognitive performances of nondemented participants have also been reported in several RCTs,[46–50] although others found no cognitive improvement in physically active groups.[41,51–53] Most of these RCTs were based on small samples of young-old participants, and were short-term trials, none of which were designed to assess incidence of AD or dementia as the main outcome. These RCTs concluded that compared with controls, individuals assigned to a physical exercise program improved[48,51–56] or maintained[57] their cognitive function. In a young-old population, Molloy and colleagues[58] also suggested that the acute effects of an exercise program on neuropsychological function were not long-lasting.

Other small RCTs, in elderly people living in the community or in nursing-home residents, have failed to show any improvement of cognitive function.[47,55,57,59–64] One explanation may be that most exercise programs last a few months, whereas physical activity may protect cognitive function in the long-term.

Colcombe and Kramer[65] in 2003 performed a meta-analysis of 18 interventional studies published between 1966 and 2001 and reported a significant but selective

Table 1
Observational studies of physical activity and risk of AD or dementia

Author and Study Name	Longitudinal Nondemented Population-Based Study	Summary of Major Findings (Adjusted for Confounders)
Li et al[10]	1090 individuals aged 60 years or more	Individuals with limited physical activity had a higher risk for developing dementia
Stern et al[11]	593 individuals aged 60 years or more	Individuals with low lifetime occupational attainment had a higher risk for developing dementia (RR 2.25, 95% CI 1.32–3.84)
Yoshitake et al[12] Hisayama Study	828 individuals aged 65 years or more	Physical activity was a significant preventive factor for AD
Fabrigoule et al[13] Paquid Study	2040 individuals aged 65 years or more	Physically active individuals had a lower risk of dementia (RR 0.33, 95% CI 0.10–1.04)
Broe et al[14] Sydney Older Persons Study	327 individuals aged 75 years or more	No statistically significant association between physical activity and dementia
Laurin et al[15] Canadian Study of Health and Aging	6434 individuals aged 65 years or more	High levels of physical activity were associated with reduced risks of cognitive impairment (OR 0.58, 95% CI 0.41–0.83), AD (OR 0.50, 95% CI 0.28–0.90), and dementia of any type (OR 0.63, 95% CI 0.40–0.98)
Scarmeas et al[16] Health Care Financing Administration Study	1772 individuals aged 65 years or more	Subjects with high leisure activities (RR 0.62, 95% CI 0.46–0.83) Walking for pleasure or going on an excursion (RR 0.73, 95% CI 0.55–0.98)
Ho et al[17]	2030 individuals aged 70 years or more	Sedentary behavior was associated with an increased risk of cognitive impairment
Lindsay et al[15] Canadian Study of Health and Aging	6434 individuals aged 65 years or more	Regular physical activity was associated with a reduced risk of AD (OR 0.69, 95% CI 0.5–0.96)

Study	Population	Findings
Wang et al[18] Kungsholmen Project	776 individuals aged 75 years or more	Daily physical activity was associated with no significant reduction in risk of dementia (RR 0.41, 95% CI 0.13–1.31)
Yamada et al[19] Radiation Effect Research Foundation Adult Health Study	1774 individuals	No statistically significant association between physical activity and dementia
Verghese et al[20] Bronx Aging Study	469 individuals aged 75 years or more	Leisure cognitive activities were associated with a reduced risk of dementia but physical activity was not. Dancing was the only physical activity associated with a lower risk of dementia (HR 0.24, 95% CI 0.06–0.99)
Abbott et al[21] Honolulu-Asia Aging Study	2257 men aged 71–93 years	Men who walked less than 0.25 miles/d experienced a 1.8-fold excess risk of dementia compared with those who walked more than 2 miles/d (HR 1.77, 95% CI 1.04–3.01)
Podewils et al[22] Cardiovascular Health Cognitive Study	3375 individuals aged 65 years or more	Individuals in the highest quartile of physical energy expenditure had lower risk of dementia (RR 0.85, 95% CI 0.61–1.19) compared with those in the lowest quartile; individuals engaging in more than 4 activities had lower risk of dementia (RR 0.51, 95% CI 0.33–0.79) compared with those engaging in 0–1 activity
Rovio et al[23] Cardiovascular risk factors, Aging and Incidence of Dementia (CAIDE)	1449 individuals aged 65–79 years	Leisure-time physical activity, at least twice a week, was associated with a reduced risk of dementia and AD (OR 0.48, 95% CI 0.25–0.91 and 0.38, 95% CI 0.17–0.85, respectively)
Larson et al[24] Adult Change in Thought	1740 individuals aged 65 years or more	Active (more than 3 times/wk) compared with fewer than 3 times/wk (HR 0.68, 95% CI 0.48–0.96 for dementia and 0.69, 95% CI 0.45–1.05 for AD)

Abbreviations: CI, confidence interval; HR, hazard ratio; OR, odds ratio; RR, relative risk.

Table 2
Observational studies of physical activity and risk of cognitive decline

Author and Study Name	Longitudinal Nondemented Population-Based Study	Summary of Major Findings (Adjusted for Confounders)
Albert et al[25] MacArthur Study	1192 individuals aged 70–79 years	Strenuous physical activity but not moderate physical activity was associated with a reduced risk of cognitive decline
Broe et al[14] Sydney Older Persons Study	327 individuals aged 75 years or more	No statistically significant association between physical activity and cognitive decline
Schuit et al[26]	347 individuals aged 65 years or more	Low physical activity group had a 2-fold risk of cognitive decline (OR 2.0, 95% CI 0.9–4.8)
Yaffe et al[27] Study of Osteoporotic Fractures	5925 individuals aged 65 years or more	Highest quartile compared with the lowest quartile of blocks walked (OR 0.66, 95% CI 0.54–0.82)
Pignatti et al[28] Brescia Study	364 individuals aged 70–85 years	Inactivity was associated with a higher risk of cognitive decline (RR 3.7, 95% CI 1.2–11.1)
Dik et al[29]	1241 individuals aged 62–85 years	Active men at low or moderate level displayed faster processing speed
Barnes et al[30] Sonoma study	349 individuals aged 55 years or more	Cognitive decline is associated with baseline peak oxygen consumption (VO_2) Lowest VO_2 tertile = -0.5 (-0.8 to 0.3)/middle VO_2 tertile = -0.2 (-0.5 to 0.0)/highest VO_2 tertile = 0.0 (-0.3 to 0.2) $P = .002$ for trend over tertiles
Lytle et al[31] Monongahela Valley Independent Elders Survey (MoVIES)	1146 individuals aged 65 years or more	High exercise (OR 0.39, 95% CI 0.19–0.78) Threshold = 5 times/wk
Weuve et al[32] Nurses' Health Study	18,766 women aged 70–81 years	Women in the highest quintile of activity had lower cognitive decline (OR 0.80, 95% CI 0.67–0.95) Walking at least 1.5 hours/wk at a pace of 21–30 min/mile was associated with a significantly higher cognitive score

effect of fitness training on cognitive function, with the main benefits occurring in executive-control processes. In 2006, the same investigators[66] reported a significant increase in brain volume in volunteers aged 60 to 79 years who participated in a 6-month aerobic program. Their findings provide convincing support for the hypothesis that physical activity prevents age-related cognitive decline.

In 2008, Lautenschlager and colleagues[8] published the first trial to show that a physical activity program (about 20 min/d) modestly improved the cognitive function of 170 older adults with subjective and objective mild cognitive impairment. An average improvement of 1.3 points on the Alzheimer's Disease Assessment Scale-Cognitive Subscale (ADAS-cog) relative to the usual care control group after 6 months and 0.69 points at 18 months was reported. These results compare favorably with the benefit reported with the use of donepezil.[67] Recently, Williamson and colleagues[7] reported the results from the cognitive substudy of the Lifestyle Interventions and Independence for Elders pilot (LIFE-P) study. In this RCT pilot study, 102 older adults at risk for mobility disability participated in a physical activity intervention for 1 year. The investigators reported a significant correlation between physical and cognitive performance.

In a recent Cochrane review Angevaren and colleagues[68] assessed the effectiveness of physical activity on cognitive function in people older than 55 years without cognitive impairment. Eight of 11 RCTs that compared aerobic physical activity programs with any other intervention or no intervention reported an improvement in cognitive capacity that coincided with the increased cardiorespiratory fitness of the intervention group. The largest effects on cognitive function were found on motor function and auditory attention. The investigators reported an effect size of 1.17 for the motor function and 0.50 for auditory attention, which were the cognitive domains with the largest effects. For cognitive speed and visual attention, a moderate effect was observed, with an effect size of 0.26 for both domains.

Larger studies are still required to increase knowledge regarding the relationship between exercise and cognitive function in humans. However, most RCTs of physical activity in older adults suggest a selective improvement in executive control processes.[53,68] Aerobic exercise intervention enhances executive function, although other cognitive functions seem to be insensitive to physical exercise (aerobic exercise affected cognitive and neural plasticity in a cross-sectional study).[51]

The specificity that aerobic exercise has on executive function suggests some specificity for aerobic exercise on brain function that requires further research.[68] Research on neuroimaging suggests that prefrontal and parietal circuits in the brain, the regions of the brain that are most involved in executive control, retain more plasticity. For example, in a cross-sectional study, Colcombe and colleagues[69] reported that fitter older subjects had a greater volume of gray matter in the prefrontal, parietal, and temporal regions and a greater volume of white matter in the genu of the corpus callosum than their less fit counterparts, after controlling for potential confounders.

Epidemiologic studies have also reported that low physical performance[70-72] is associated with higher rates of cognitive decline and dementia. Low physical activity is 1 of the main factors for poor physical performance. A poor score on tests such as walking speed,[70-72] or poor results on the timed chair-stand test, standing balance, or grip-strength tests,[72] are associated with higher rates of cognitive decline and dementia. In cross-sectional studies, cardiovascular fitness was associated with attention and executive function[73,74] or visuospatial function.[75] In the Sydney Older Person Study, participants with cognitive impairment and slow gait were most likely to progress to dementia during a 6-year period.[76] The REAL FR study reported that an abnormal 1-leg balance predicts higher rate of cognitive decline.[77] On the other hand, during the 7-year follow-up of the Hispanic Established Population for the Epidemiologic Study of the Elderly (EPESE), participants with poor cognition had a steeper decline in physical performance than those with good cognition.[78] These results reinforced the growing evidence of the links between physical performance and cognition.

Basic Research

Numerous studies on rodents suggested that exercise improves acquisition and retention in memory-dependent tasks such as the radial arm maze,[79] the Morris water maze,[80,81] passive avoidance,[82] and object recognition.[83] There is no clear explanation for this relation between physical activity and brain function. However, numerous hypotheses have been put forward and growing evidence from animal research suggests that physical activity may directly modulate the formation of β-amyloid protein through several biologic mechanisms. A review published in 2007 by Cotman and colleagues[84] examined the multiple underlying mechanisms promoted by physical activity to ensure brain health. One hypothesis is an improvement in cerebral vascular functioning and brain perfusion. Animal[85] and human[86] studies have shown that physical activity can stimulate brain perfusion and angiogenesis within a few weeks of aerobic training. Physical activity is associated with increased blood perfusion of brain regions that modulate attention. The common pathway of the other mechanisms involved may be a preventive effect of physical activity on the inflammatory pathway and its deleterious consequences on growth factor signaling.[84] These effects may be mediated by activation of insulinlike growth factor 1, vascular endothelial growth factor, brain-derived neurotrophic factor, and endorphins. The neurotrophin brain-derived neurotrophic factor is considered to be the most important factor upregulated by physical activity. It has an important role in cell genesis and growth. The synaptogenesis, neurogenesis, and attenuation of neural responses to stress stimulated by physical activity explain brain plasticity.[87,88] These mechanisms may also enhance brain cytoarchitecture and electrophysiologic properties, suggesting that the brain retains the capacity to regenerate new connections and new neurons. An external stimulus such as physical activity may influence the age-related neurologic process or the neuropathological AD processes. Participation in physical activity may thus lower the risk of cognitive decline and dementia by improving cognitive reserve.[13,15,16,18,50,89,90]

Higher cognitive reserve may help the subject engage in regular physical activity to cope with the first cognitive symptoms of AD. This effect may delay the onset of the clinical manifestations of the disease, which may become apparent only later. The recent basic research has yielded convincing arguments that physical activity acts as a stimulus of neurogenesis, enhances the brain cytoarchitecture and electrophysiologic properties, and may influence neuropathologic processes such as the formation of β-amyloid protein during AD.

With a view to preventing cognitive decline, dementia, and AD, it remains unclear how much physical activity, what type, and at what time of lifespan, is optimally effective in preventing cognitive decline and dementia. Although conclusive evidence is lacking to answer these questions, epidemiologic and animal studies suggest the conditions (intensity, type, frequency, and duration) under which physical activity may reduce the risk of dementia. It also remains to be determined whether voluntary and forced exercise result in the same improvement.

SUMMARY

Regular physical activity is a key component of successful aging. Increasing evidence suggests that an active life has a protective effect on brain functioning in the elderly population. Epidemiologic studies, short-term RCTs in nondemented participants, and biologic research suggest that physical activity improves cognitive functioning in older subjects. However, no RCT has yet shown that regular physical activity prevents dementia. Additional interventional studies are needed to examine this relationship. Moreover, type, duration, and intensity of physical exercise, and its precise impact on the different aspects of cognitive function, need to be determined in RCTs. Future research should focus on developing specific exercise programs to postpone or reduce the risk of dementia, or slow down disease progression. In the coming decade, large ongoing RCTs may provide some of the answers to these questions. Preventive approaches to dementia could then be the basis of recommendations to the community. The main challenge, however, is how to change lifestyle habits and promote physical activity in the older population in the long-term. In primary care, prevention of many diseases already relies on a healthy diet and lifestyle, control of cardiovascular risk factors, ongoing learning experiences, and regular physical activity. Prevention of cognitive decline and dementia could be a decisive argument to convince patients and modify public health policy.

REFERENCES

1. Physical activity and cardiovascular health. NIH Consensus Development Panel on Physical Activity and Cardiovascular Health. JAMA 1996;276(3):241–6.
2. Thune I, Furberg AS. Physical activity and cancer risk: dose-response and cancer, all sites and site-specific. Med Sci Sports Exerc 2001;33(Suppl 6): S530–50 [discussion: S609–10].
3. Brody JG, Rudel RA, Michels KB, et al. Environmental pollutants, diet, physical activity, body size, and breast cancer: where do we stand in research to identify opportunities for prevention? Cancer 2007;109(Suppl 12):2627–34.
4. Fratiglioni L, Winblad B, von Strauss E. Prevention of Alzheimer's disease and dementia. Major findings from the Kungsholmen project. Physiol Behav 2007; 92(1–2):98–104.
5. Kawas CH, Brookmeyer R. Aging and the public health effects of dementia. N Engl J Med 2001;344(15):1160–1.
6. Coley N, Andrieu S, Gardette V, et al. Dementia prevention: methodological explanations for inconsistent results. Epidemiol Rev 2008;30:35–66.
7. Williamson JD, Espeland M, Kritchevsky SB, et al. Changes in cognitive function in a randomized trial of physical activity: results of the lifestyle interventions and independence for elders pilot study. J Gerontol A Biol Sci Med Sci 2009;64(6): 688–94.
8. Lautenschlager NT, Cox KL, Flicker L, et al. Effect of physical activity on cognitive function in older adults at risk for Alzheimer disease: a randomized trial. JAMA 2008;300(9):1027–37.
9. Rolland Y, Abellan van Kan G, Vellas B. Physical activity and Alzheimer's disease: from prevention to therapeutic perspectives. J Am Med Dir Assoc 2008;9(6): 390–405.
10. Li G, Shen YC, Chen CH, et al. A three-year follow-up study of age-related dementia in an urban area of Beijing. Acta Psychiatr Scand 1991;83(2):99–104.
11. Stern Y, Gurland B, Tatemichi TK, et al. Influence of education and occupation on the incidence of Alzheimer's disease. JAMA 1994;271(13):1004–10.
12. Yoshitake T, Kiyohara Y, Kato I, et al. Incidence and risk factors of vascular dementia and Alzheimer's disease in a defined elderly Japanese population: the Hisayama Study. Neurology 1995;45(6):1161–8.

13. Fabrigoule C, Letenneur L, Dartigues JF, et al. Social and leisure activities and risk of dementia: a prospective longitudinal study. J Am Geriatr Soc 1995; 43(5):485–90.
14. Broe GA, Creasey H, Jorm AF, et al. Health habits and risk of cognitive impairment and dementia in old age: a prospective study on the effects of exercise, smoking and alcohol consumption. Aust N Z J Public Health 1998;22(5):621–3.
15. Laurin D, Verreault R, Lindsay J, et al. Physical activity and risk of cognitive impairment and dementia in elderly persons. Arch Neurol 2001;58(3):498–504.
16. Scarmeas N, Levy G, Tang MX, et al. Influence of leisure activity on the incidence of Alzheimer's disease. Neurology 2001;57(12):2236–42.
17. Ho SC, Woo J, Sham A, et al. A 3-year follow-up study of social, lifestyle and health predictors of cognitive impairment in a Chinese older cohort. Int J Epidemiol 2001;30(6):1389–96.
18. Wang HX, Karp A, Winblad B, et al. Late-life engagement in social and leisure activities is associated with a decreased risk of dementia: a longitudinal study from the Kungsholmen project. Am J Epidemiol 2002;155(12):1081–7.
19. Yamada M, Kasagi F, Sasaki H, et al. Association between dementia and midlife risk factors: the Radiation Effects Research Foundation Adult Health Study. J Am Geriatr Soc 2003;51(3):410–4.
20. Verghese J, Lipton RB, Katz MJ, et al. Leisure activities and the risk of dementia in the elderly. N Engl J Med 2003;348(25):2508–16.
21. Abbott RD, White LR, Ross GW, et al. Walking and dementia in physically capable elderly men. JAMA 2004;292(12):1447–53.
22. Podewils LJ, Guallar E, Kuller LH, et al. Physical activity, APOE genotype, and dementia risk: findings from the Cardiovascular Health Cognition Study. Am J Epidemiol 2005;161(7):639–51.
23. Rovio S, Kareholt I, Helkala EL, et al. Leisure-time physical activity at midlife and the risk of dementia and Alzheimer's disease. Lancet Neurol 2005;4(11):705–11.
24. Larson EB, Wang L, Bowen JD, et al. Exercise is associated with reduced risk for incident dementia among persons 65 years of age and older. Ann Intern Med 2006;144(2):73–81.
25. Albert MS, Jones K, Savage CR, et al. Predictors of cognitive change in older persons: MacArthur studies of successful aging. Psychol Aging 1995;10(4):578–89.
26. Schuit AJ, Feskens EJ, Launer LJ, et al. Physical activity and cognitive decline, the role of the apolipoprotein e4 allele. Med Sci Sports Exerc 2001;33(5):772–7.
27. Yaffe K, Barnes D, Nevitt M, et al. A prospective study of physical activity and cognitive decline in elderly women: women who walk. Arch Intern Med 2001; 161(14):1703–8.
28. Pignatti F, Rozzini R, Trabucchi M. Physical activity and cognitive decline in elderly persons. Arch Intern Med 2002;162(3):361–2.
29. Dik M, Deeg DJ, Visser M, et al. Early life physical activity and cognition at old age. J Clin Exp Neuropsychol 2003;25(5):643–53.
30. Barnes DE, Yaffe K, Satariano WA, et al. A longitudinal study of cardiorespiratory fitness and cognitive function in healthy older adults. J Am Geriatr Soc 2003;51(4):459–65.
31. Lytle ME, Vander Bilt J, Pandav RS, et al. Exercise level and cognitive decline: the MoVIES project. Alzheimer Dis Assoc Disord 2004;18(2):57–64.
32. Weuve J, Kang JH, Manson JE, et al. Physical activity, including walking, and cognitive function in older women. JAMA 2004;292(12):1454–61.
33. Aguero-Torres H, Fratiglioni L, Guo Z, et al. Dementia is the major cause of functional dependence in the elderly: 3-year follow-up data from a population-based study. Am J Public Health 1998;88(10):1452–6.

34. Wang L, van Belle G, Kukull WB, et al. Predictors of functional change: a longitudinal study of nondemented people aged 65 and older. J Am Geriatr Soc 2002; 50(9):1525–34.
35. Moritz DJ, Kasl SV, Berkman LF. Cognitive functioning and the incidence of limitations in activities of daily living in an elderly community sample. Am J Epidemiol 1995;141(1):41–9.
36. Korczyn AD, Halperin I. Depression and dementia. J Neurol Sci 2009;283(1–2): 139–42.
37. Smyth KA, Fritsch T, Cook TB, et al. Worker functions and traits associated with occupations and the development of AD. Neurology 2004;63(3):498–503.
38. McKhann G, Drachman D, Folstein M, et al. Clinical diagnosis of Alzheimer's disease: report of the NINCDS-ADRDA Work Group under the auspices of Department of Health and Human Services Task Force on Alzheimer's Disease. Neurology 1984;34(7):939–44.
39. Broe GA, Henderson AS, Creasey H, et al. A case-control study of Alzheimer's disease in Australia. Neurology 1990;40(11):1698–707.
40. Christensen H, Korten A, Jorm AF, et al. Activity levels and cognitive functioning in an elderly community sample. Age Ageing 1996;25(1):72–80.
41. Emery CF, Schein RL, Hauck ER, et al. Psychological and cognitive outcomes of a randomized trial of exercise among patients with chronic obstructive pulmonary disease. Health Psychol 1998;17(3):232–40.
42. Clarkson-Smith L, Hartley AA. Relationships between physical exercise and cognitive abilities in older adults. Psychol Aging 1989;4(2):183–9.
43. Carmelli D, Swan GE, LaRue A, et al. Correlates of change in cognitive function in survivors from the Western Collaborative Group Study. Neuroepidemiology 1997; 16(6):285–95.
44. Friedland RP, Fritsch T, Smyth KA, et al. Patients with Alzheimer's disease have reduced activities in midlife compared with healthy control-group members. Proc Natl Acad Sci U S A 2001;98(6):3440–5.
45. Hultsch DF, Hammer M, Small BJ. Age differences in cognitive performance in later life: relationships to self-reported health and activity life style. J Gerontol 1993;48(1):P1–11.
46. Pierce TW, Madden DJ, Siegel WC, et al. Effects of aerobic exercise on cognitive and psychosocial functioning in patients with mild hypertension. Health Psychol 1993;12(4):286–91.
47. Madden DJ, Blumenthal JA, Allen PA, et al. Improving aerobic capacity in healthy older adults does not necessarily lead to improved cognitive performance. Psychol Aging 1989;4(3):307–20.
48. Blumenthal JA, Emery CF, Madden DJ, et al. Long-term effects of exercise on psychological functioning in older men and women. J Gerontol 1991;46(6): P352–61.
49. Emery CF, Huppert FA, Schein RL. Relationships among age, exercise, health, and cognitive function in a British sample. Gerontologist 1995;35(3):378–85.
50. Rogers RL, Meyer JS, Mortel KF. After reaching retirement age physical activity sustains cerebral perfusion and cognition. J Am Geriatr Soc 1990; 38(2):123–8.
51. Dustman RE, Ruhling RO, Russell EM, et al. Aerobic exercise training and improved neuropsychological function of older individuals. Neurobiol Aging 1984;5(1):35–42.
52. Williams P, Lord SR. Effects of group exercise on cognitive functioning and mood in older women. Aust N Z J Public Health 1997;21(1):45–52.

53. Kramer AF, Hahn S, Cohen NJ, et al. Ageing, fitness and neurocognitive function. Nature 1999;400(6743):418–9.
54. Hassmen P, Koivula N. Mood, physical working capacity and cognitive performance in the elderly as related to physical activity. Aging (Milano) 1997;9(1–2):136–42.
55. Emery CF, Gatz M. Psychological and cognitive effects of an exercise program for community-residing older adults. Gerontologist 1990;30(2):184–8.
56. Fabre C, Chamari K, Mucci P, et al. Improvement of cognitive function by mental and/or individualized aerobic training in healthy elderly subjects. Int J Sports Med 2002;23(6):415–21.
57. Hill RD, Storandt M, Malley M. The impact of long-term exercise training on psychological function in older adults. J Gerontol 1993;48(1):P12–7.
58. Molloy DW, Beerschoten DA, Borrie MJ, et al. Acute effects of exercise on neuropsychological function in elderly subjects. J Am Geriatr Soc 1988;36(1):29–33.
59. Molloy DW, Richardson LD, Crilly RG. The effects of a three-month exercise programme on neuropsychological function in elderly institutionalized women: a randomized controlled trial. Age Ageing 1988;17(5):303–10.
60. Thompson RF, Crist DM, Marsh M, et al. Effects of physical exercise for elderly patients with physical impairments. J Am Geriatr Soc 1988;36(2):130–5.
61. Barry AJ, Steinmetz JR, Page HF, et al. The effects of physical conditioning on older individuals. II. Motor performance and cognitive function. J Gerontol 1966;21(2):192–9.
62. Blumenthal JA, Emery CF, Madden DJ, et al. Cardiovascular and behavioral effects of aerobic exercise training in healthy older men and women. J Gerontol 1989;44(5):M147–57.
63. Okumiya K, Matsubayashi K, Wada T, et al. Effects of exercise on neurobehavioral function in community-dwelling older people more than 75 years of age. J Am Geriatr Soc 1996;44(5):569–72.
64. Stevenson JS, Topp R. Effects of moderate and low intensity long-term exercise by older adults. Res Nurs Health 1990;13(4):209–18.
65. Colcombe S, Kramer AF. Fitness effects on the cognitive function of older adults: a meta-analytic study. Psychol Sci 2003;14(2):125–30.
66. Colcombe SJ, Erickson KI, Scalf PE, et al. Aerobic exercise training increases brain volume in aging humans. J Gerontol A Biol Sci Med Sci 2006;61(11):1166–70.
67. Petersen RC, Thomas RG, Grundman M, et al. Vitamin E and donepezil for the treatment of mild cognitive impairment. N Engl J Med 2005;352(23):2379–88.
68. Angevaren M, Aufdemkampe G, Verhaar HJ, et al. Physical activity and enhanced fitness to improve cognitive function in older people without known cognitive impairment. Cochrane Database Syst Rev 2008;(3):CD005381.
69. Colcombe SJ, Erickson KI, Raz N, et al. Aerobic fitness reduces brain tissue loss in aging humans. J Gerontol A Biol Sci Med Sci 2003;58(2):176–80.
70. Camicioli R, Howieson D, Oken B, et al. Motor slowing precedes cognitive impairment in the oldest old. Neurology 1998;50(5):1496–8.
71. Marquis S, Moore MM, Howieson DB, et al. Independent predictors of cognitive decline in healthy elderly persons. Arch Neurol 2002;59(4):601–6.
72. Wang L, Larson EB, Bowen JD, et al. Performance-based physical function and future dementia in older people. Arch Intern Med 2006;166(10):1115–20.
73. Dustman RE, Emmerson RY, Ruhling RO, et al. Age and fitness effects on EEG, ERPs, visual sensitivity, and cognition. Neurobiol Aging 1990;11(3):193–200.
74. van Boxtel MP, Paas FG, Houx PJ, et al. Aerobic capacity and cognitive performance in a cross-sectional aging study. Med Sci Sports Exerc 1997;29(10):1357–65.

75. Shay KA, Roth DL. Association between aerobic fitness and visuospatial performance in healthy older adults. Psychol Aging 1992;7(1):15–24.
76. Waite LM, Grayson DA, Piguet O, et al. Gait slowing as a predictor of incident dementia: 6-year longitudinal data from the Sydney Older Persons Study. J Neurol Sci 2005;229-230:89–93.
77. Rolland Y, Abellan van Kan G, Nourhashemi F, et al. An abnormal "one-leg balance" test predicts cognitive decline during Alzheimer's disease. J Alzheimers Dis 2009;16(3):525–31.
78. Raji MA, Kuo YF, Snih SA, et al. Cognitive status, muscle strength, and subsequent disability in older Mexican Americans. J Am Geriatr Soc 2005;53(9):1462–8.
79. Schweitzer NB, Alessio HM, Berry SD, et al. Exercise-induced changes in cardiac gene expression and its relation to spatial maze performance. Neurochem Int 2006;48(1):9–16.
80. van Praag H, Shubert T, Zhao C, et al. Exercise enhances learning and hippocampal neurogenesis in aged mice. J Neurosci 2005;25(38):8680–5.
81. Vaynman S, Ying Z, Gomez-Pinilla F. Hippocampal BDNF mediates the efficacy of exercise on synaptic plasticity and cognition. Eur J Neurosci 2004;20(10):2580–90.
82. Radak Z, Toldy A, Szabo Z, et al. The effects of training and detraining on memory, neurotrophins and oxidative stress markers in rat brain. Neurochem Int 2006;49(4):387–92.
83. O'Callaghan RM, Ohle R, Kelly AM. The effects of forced exercise on hippocampal plasticity in the rat: a comparison of LTP, spatial- and non-spatial learning. Behav Brain Res 2007;176(2):362–6.
84. Cotman CW, Berchtold NC, Christie LA. Exercise builds brain health: key roles of growth factor cascades and inflammation. Trends Neurosci 2007;30(9):464–72.
85. Swain RA, Harris AB, Wiener EC, et al. Prolonged exercise induces angiogenesis and increases cerebral blood volume in primary motor cortex of the rat. Neuroscience 2003;117(4):1037–46.
86. Colcombe SJ, Kramer AF, Erickson KI, et al. Cardiovascular fitness, cortical plasticity, and aging. Proc Natl Acad Sci U S A 2004;101(9):3316–21.
87. Kronenberg G, Bick-Sander A, Bunk E, et al. Physical exercise prevents age-related decline in precursor cell activity in the mouse dentate gyrus. Neurobiol Aging 2006;27(10):1505–13.
88. Uda M, Ishido M, Kami K, et al. Effects of chronic treadmill running on neurogenesis in the dentate gyrus of the hippocampus of adult rat. Brain Res 2006;1104(1):64–72.
89. Wilson RS, Mendes De Leon CF, Barnes LL, et al. Participation in cognitively stimulating activities and risk of incident Alzheimer disease. JAMA 2002;287(6):742–8.
90. Wilson RS, Bennett DA, Bienias JL, et al. Cognitive activity and incident AD in a population-based sample of older persons. Neurology 2002;59(12):1910–4.

Nutrition and the Brain

John E. Morley, MB, BCh[a,b,*]

KEYWORDS

- Nutrition • Brain • Triglycerides • Leptin
- Lutein • Alpha-lipoic acid

Food is essential for all the functions of the body, and this is especially true of the brain. Protein energy malnutrition is associated with poor cognition.[1–4] Historically, vitamin deficiencies have been associated with severe cognitive problems, such as nicotinamide deficiency leading to pellagra and thiamine deficiency leading to Wernicke encephalopathy. Multiple vitamin deficiencies have been associated with delirium, the 6th vital sign.[5–7]

Dementia is a major cause of frailty and disability in older persons.[8–10] It has been shown that exercise prevents the development of Alzheimer disease[11–13] and slows the deterioration seen in patients with established dementia.[14–16] Although the role of nutrition is less clear, emerging evidence supports that certain nutrients can be equally effective in playing a role in the prevention of dementia. This article discusses the emerging area of the role of nutrition in producing cognitive disturbances.

THE GUT-BRAIN AXIS

Several years ago the author showed that feeding an animal after it learned a task improved its ability to remember the task.[17] This was due to the release of the gastrointestinal hormone, cholecystokinin (CCK). CCK activated the ascending fibers of the vagus to send messages to the nucleus tractus solitarius and from there to the amygdale and the hippocampus.[18,19]

The author has found that the stomach hormone, ghrelin, which is elevated during starvation, is responsible for restoring memories.[20] Receptors for ghrelin are in the

No external funding was received, and the author has no conflict of interest to declare regarding this work.

[a] Division of Geriatric Medicine, Saint Louis University School of Medicine, 1402 South Grand Boulevard, M238, St Louis, MO 63104, USA

[b] Geriatric Research Education and Clinical Center, Veterans Affairs Medical Center, St Louis, MO 63125, USA

* Division of Geriatric Medicine, Saint Louis University School of Medicine, 1402 South Grand Boulevard, M238, St Louis, MO 63104.

E-mail address: morley@slu.edu

Clin Geriatr Med 26 (2010) 89–98
doi:10.1016/j.cger.2009.11.005
0749-0690/10/$ – see front matter. Published by Elsevier Inc.

hippocampus. Ghrelin also enhanced recall of memories in an animal model of dementia, the SAMP8 mouse.[21–23]

The combination of CCK and ghrelin is known as the gut-brain axis[24] and plays an important role in allowing animals to successfully forage for food (**Fig. 1**).

FAT-BRAIN AXIS

Leptin is a peptide hormone that is produced by adipocytes. Leptin enhances memory.[25] As leptin is produced by fat cells, it provides one of the mechanisms by which malnutrition can lead to decreased cognition (**Fig. 2**).

Some obese persons have problems with learning. The mechanism for this was uncertain until recently. The author found that memory problems were associated with hypertriglyceridemia. Triglycerides interfered with long-term potentiation, the electrical equivalent of memory.[26] Lowering triglycerides with a peroxisome proliferator-activated receptor–alpha agent, gemfibrozil, resulted in improved memory. Triglycerides inhibit the ability of leptin to cross the blood-brain barrier.[27] Thus, triglycerides decrease learning and memory by inhibiting the effects of leptin on the hippocampus.

Elevated triglyceride levels were shown to be associated with delirium. Lower levels of hypertriglyceridemia produce mild cognitive deficits.[28,29] These deficits can be reversed by lowering the triglyceride levels.

DIABETES MELLITUS AND MEMORY

It has been shown that hypoglycemia leads to delirium.[30] It is recognized that hyperglycemia also leads to cognitive problems.[31,32] These memory problems can be reversed by lowering the glucose levels to the normal range.[33]

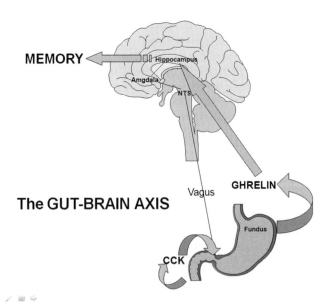

Fig. 1. The gut-brain axis. CCK activates ascending fibers in the vagus going to the nucleus tractus solitarius (NTS). Fibers from the NTS activate the amygdale and hippocampus to enhance storage of memories. Ghrelin from the fundus of the stomach activates hippocampal neurons to facilitate retrieval of memories.

The Fat-Brain Axis

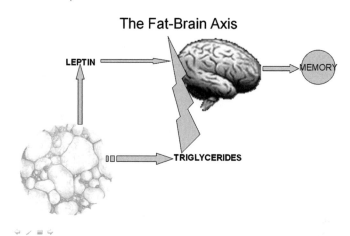

Fig. 2. The fat-brain axis. Leptin activates neurons in the hippocampus to store memories. Triglycerides inhibit leptin from crossing the blood-brain barrier, and this inhibits memory formation.

Persons with chronic hyperglycemia are at a risk for developing atherosclerosis.[34,35] Over time, this can lead to multiple small infarcts in the brain, which eventually cause vascular dementia. Thus, it is not surprising that persons with diabetes mellitus are more likely to develop dementia.

Persons with diabetes are more likely to have depression.[36] When depression is coupled with hyperglycemia, it is common to see poor compliance in diabetic individuals.[37] This can particularly be a problem in older persons, in whom mild cognitive impairment is common. This makes it essential to screen all patients with diabetes mellitus for mild cognitive impairment, using sensitive tools such as the Veterans Administration-Saint Louis University Mental Status (SLUMS) Examination.[38–40]

The role of insulin in memory regulation is less clear. Insulin degrading enzyme also degrades amyloid-β protein,[41] suggesting that insulin could be associated with an increase in amyloid-β protein and, therefore, with a decline in cognition. However, recently it was found that low concentrations of amyloid-β protein is actually a physiologic enhancer of memory.[42] Some studies have suggested that intranasal insulin enhances memory, supporting this concept.[43]

VITAMIN B$_{12}$ DEFICIENCY

Vitamin B$_{12}$ deficiency is classically on the list of reversible dementia.[44] In its full-blown manifestation, as pernicious anemia, it presents with megaloblastic anemia, dementia, and a posterior column neuropathy (loss of vibration and position sense). However, vitamin B$_{12}$ deficiency can present as a dementia without any of the other features.

Assays for vitamin B$_{12}$ deficiency do not display a high level of accuracy. For this reason, when a person has a low normal vitamin B$_{12}$ level, further testing needs to be done. This involves measuring homocysteine and methylmalonic acid levels. If both are elevated, it suggests that the person has vitamin B$_{12}$ deficiency, whereas if only homocysteine is elevated, it suggests folate deficiency. Folate deficiency is also associated with poor cognition.

VITAMIN D DEFICIENCY

One of the greatest public health successes of the last 30 years has been to convince people to protect their skin from the sun by using sunblock. This has led to an epidemic of vitamin D deficiency with more than two-thirds of young children being vitamin D deficient and almost every older person in a nursing home suffering the same fate.[45–48] Perry and colleagues[49] found that in the whole population of older persons, vitamin D decreased over a 14-year period. Older persons have a decreased production of cholecalciferol in their skin and a decreased absorption of vitamin D in the gastrointestinal tract.

Well-recognized effects of vitamin D deficiency include hip fractures, falls, functional deterioration, muscle pain, and increased mortality.[50] It is now recognized that deficiency of 25-hydroxy (OH) vitamin D is associated with cognitive impairment.[51–54] For these reasons, it is essential to measure 25-OH vitamin D levels. Vitamin D replacement needs to be performed if the level is below 30 ng/ml.

FREE RADICALS AND OXIDATIVE DAMAGE

A major theory of Alzheimer disease is that amyloid-β protein activates free radicals in the brain, leading to oxidative damage and destruction of neurons.[55] This has lead to the attempt to slow the progress of Alzheimer disease by using the free radical scavanger, vitamin E.[56] However, the outcomes of these studies have been disappointing.

Alpha-lipoic acid is a more powerful free radical scavenger than is vitamin E. The SAMP8 mouse is a model of overproduction of amyloid-β protein, which is associated with severe oxidative damage of the brain that is associated with learning and memory problems occurring between 8 to 12 months of age.[57–63] In this animal model, the author has shown that alpha-lipoic acid not only improves memory but also markedly reduces free radical damage in the brain.[62,64] Alpha-lipoic acid has improved cognitive performance in also other mouse models of dementia.[65–68]

In humans, alpha-lipoic acid has been shown to markedly improve diabetic peripheral neuropathy.[69] Besides its antioxidant activities alpha-lipoic acid also increases endothelial nitric oxide synthase activity, activates phase 2 detoxification, and limits the expression of nuclear factor (NF) κB activity.[70] Limiting NF-κB activity decreases cytokine activation. Cytokines clearly produce memory problems [71] and are associated with memory and functional decline in older persons.[72]

Hager and colleagues[73] reported a 48-month follow-up of 430 patients with Alzheimer dementia. The patients received 600 mg of alpha-lipoic acid. Patients did better than expected, but there was no placebo control arm to the study. A combination of lipoic acid and N-acetyl cysteine decreased oxidative stress and apoptotic markers in patients with Alzheimer disease.[68] The author has offered his patients with dementia the option of taking 600 to 900 mg of alpha-lipoic acid. Several patients have done this with the impression that their disease process would be slowed down. The Cochrane Database review could not find any placebo-controlled trials to justify the use of alpha-lipoic acid in Alzheimer disease.[74]

DIETARY PATTERNS AND DEMENTIA

The 3-city study in France found that daily consumption of fruits and vegetables was associated with a decrease in all causes of dementia.[75] Fish and omega-3 rich oils also reduced incidence of dementia in persons who were apolipoprotein E (ApoE) noncarriers. Huang and colleagues[76] found in the cardiovascular health cognition study that intake of fatty fish twice a week reduced dementia, but only in ApoE noncarriers. Other studies have confirmed the association of fatty fish intake with decreasing dementia.[77,78] The author's studies in the SAMP8 mouse have confirmed the positive effect of omega-3 fatty acids on improving cognition.[79,80] Low levels of docosahexaenoic acid (DHA) have been found in persons with dementia.[81]

Joseph and colleagues[82,83] have used animal studies to show that polyphenols isolated from blueberries have positive effects on dementia. They believe that this may explain the dietary fruit and vegetable data.

Curcumin, the active ingredient of curry spices, has antioxidant and antiamyloid activity.[84,85] Ng and colleagues[86] studied 1010 elderly Asians aged 60 to 93 years. They found evidence suggesting that high curry consumption was associated with improved thought processes.

Several studies have supported the concept that the Mediterranean diet may slow the progression to dementia.[87,88] Studies in SAMP8 mice support the concept that extra-virgin olive oil may play a central role in slowing the process of dementia (John Morley, unpublished data, 2009).

MEMORY SHAKES

Two "memory shakes" have been developed. The first of these is Souvenaid. It consists of uridine monophosphate, choline, and omega-3 fatty acids. There are extensive animal studies supporting its potential effects on memory.[89–91] A single multinational study has been conducted. The author's team at Saint Louis University was the only group in the United States involved in the study. Preliminary analysis of

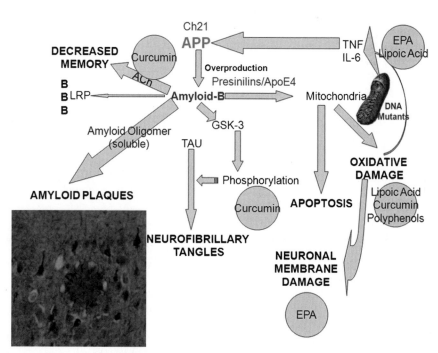

Fig. 3. Effects of nutrients to decrease the development of cognitive impairment. ACh, acetylcholine; BBB, blood-brain barrier; EPA, eicosapentaenoic acid; GSK, glycogen synthase kinase; IL-6, interleukin-6; LRP, lipoprotein receptor related peptide; TNF, tumor necrosis factor.

the study suggested that in patients with early Alzheimer disease, there was an improvement in verbal memory.

Johnson and colleagues[92] studied a combination of lutein and DHA. In their small study they found an improvement in verbal fluency, a shopping list memory test, a word list memory test, and an apartment memory test. Based on this, a new over-the-counter product for memory boosting, called Benevia, is now being marketed in the United States.

SUMMARY

Numerous nutrients have been found to improve cognition in epidemiologic and animal studies. However, there is a paucity of placebo-controlled intervention studies showing positive effects in humans. At present, vitamin D, DHA (an omega-3 fatty acid), lutein, and alpha-lipoic acid seem to have the best chance of proving to be clinically useful. The sites at which some of the nutrients affect cognition are shown in **Fig. 3**. The development of combination nutrients as "memory shakes" represents an interesting development, but has not been fully proven. None of these nutrient treatments are as efficacious as an exercise program.

REFERENCES

1. Goodwin JS, Goodwin JM, Garry PJ. Association between nutritional status and cognitive functioning in a healthy elderly population. JAMA 1983;249:2917–21.
2. Morley JE, Thomas DR. Cachexia: new advances in the management of wasting diseases. J Am Med Dir Assoc 2008;9:205–10.
3. Morley JE. Weight loss in the nursing home. J Am Med Dir Assoc 2007;8:201–4.
4. Sloane PD, Ivey J, Helton M, et al. Nutritional issues in long-term care. J Am Med Dir Assoc 2008;9:476–85.
5. Flaherty JH, Shay K, Weir C, et al. The development of a mental status vital sign for use across the spectrum of care. J Am Med Dir Assoc 2009;10:379–80.
6. Flaherty JH, Rudolph J, Shay K, et al. Delirium is a serious and under-recognized problem: why assessment of mental status should be the sixth vital sign. J Am Med Dir Assoc 2007;8:273–5.
7. Eeles E, Rockwood K. Delirium in the long-term care setting: clinical and research challenges. J Am Med Dir Assoc 2008;9:157–61.
8. Abellan van Kan G, Roland YM, Morley JE, et al. Frailty: toward a clinical definition. J Am Med Dir Assoc 2008;9:71–2.
9. Abellan van Kan G, Rolland Y, Bergman H, et al. The I.A.N.A. task force on frailty assessment of older people in clinical practice. J Nutr Health Aging 2008;12:29–37.
10. Lee M, Chodosh J. Dementia and life expectancy: what do we know? J Am Med Dir Assoc 2009;10:466–71.
11. Hogan DB, Bailey P, Black S, et al. Diagnosis and treatment of dementia: 5. Non-pharmacologic and pharmacologic therapy for mild to moderate dementia. CMAJ 2008;179:1019–26.
12. Erickson KI, Prakash RS, Voss MW, et al. Aerobic fitness is associated with hippocampal volume in elderly humans. Hippocampus 2009;19:1030–9.
13. Rolland Y, Abellan va Kan G, Vellas B. Physical activity and Alzheimer's disease: from prevention to therapeutic perspectives. J Am Med Dir Assoc 2008;9:390–405.

14. Rolland Y, Pillard F, Klapouszczak A, et al. Exercise program for nursing home residents with Alzheimer's disease: a 1-year randomized, controlled trial. J Am Geriatr Soc 2007;55:158–65.
15. Morley JE. The magic of exercise. J Am Med Dir Assoc 2008;9:375–7.
16. Morley JE. Managing persons with dementia in the nursing home: high touch trumps high tech. J Am Med Dir Assoc 2008;9:139–46.
17. Flood JF, Merbaum MO, Morley JE. The memory enhancing effects of cholecystokinin octapeptide are dependent on an intact stria terminalis. Neurobiol Learn Mem 1995;64:139–45.
18. Flood JF, Garland JS, Morley JE. Evidence that cholecystokinin-enhanced retention is mediated by changes in opioid activity in the amygdale. Brain Res 1992; 585:94–104.
19. Flood JF, Smith GE, Morley JE. Modulation of memory processing by cholecystokinin: dependence on the vagus nerve. Science 1987;236:832–4.
20. Diano S, Farr SA, Benoit SC, et al. Ghrelin controls hippocampal spine synapse density and memory performance. Nat Neurosci 2006;9:381–8.
21. Morley JE, Farr SA, Flood JF. Antibody to amyloid beta protein alleviates impaired acquisition, retention, and memory processing in SAMP8 mice. Neurobiol Learn Mem 2002;78:125–38.
22. Morley JE. The SAMP8 mouse: a model of Alzheimer disease? Biogerontology 2002;3:57–60.
23. Morley JE, Kumar VB, Bernardo AE, et al. Beta-amyloid precursor polypeptide in SAMP8 mice affects learning and memory. Peptides 2000;21:1761–7.
24. Morley JE, Flood J, Silver AJ. Effects of peripheral hormones on memory and ingestive behaviors. Psychoneuroendocrinology 1992;17:391–9.
25. Farr SA, Banks WA, Morley JE. Effects of leptin on memory processing. Peptides 2006;27:1420–5.
26. Farr SA, Yamada KA, Butterfield DA, et al. Obesity and hypertriglyceridemia produce cognitive impairment. Endocrinology 2008;149:2628–36.
27. Banks WA, Farr SA, Morley JE. The effects of high fat diets on the blood-brain barrier transport of leptin: failure or adaptation? Physiol Behav 2006;88:244–8.
28. Sims RC, Madhere S, Gordon S, et al. Relationships among blood pressure, triglycerides and verbal learning in African Americans. J Natl Med Assoc 2008; 100:1193–8.
29. De Frias CM, Bunce D, Wahlin A, et al. Cholesterol and triglycerides moderate the effect of apolipoprotein E on memory functioning in older adults. J Gerontol B Psychol Sci Soc Sci 2007;62:P112–8.
30. Mazza AD, Morley JE. Update on diabetes in the elderly and the application of current therapeutics. J Am Med Dir Assoc 2007;8:489–92.
31. Flood JF, Mooradian AD, Morley JE. Characteristics of learning and memory in streptozocin-induced diabetes mellitus. Diabetes 1990;39:1391–8.
32. Mooradian AD, Perryman K, Fitten J, et al. Cortical function in elderly non-insulin dependent diabetic patients. Behavioral and electrophysiologic studies. Arch Intern Med 1988;148:2369–72.
33. Meneilly GS, Cheung E, Tessier D, et al. The effect of improved glycemic control on cognitive functions in the elderly patient with diabetes. J Gerontol 1993;48: M117–21.
34. Strachan MW, Reynolds RM, Frier BM, et al. The relationship between type 2 diabetes and dementia. Br Med Bull 2008;88:131–46.
35. Heo JH, Lee ST, Chu Kon, et al. White matter hyperintensities and cognitive dysfunction in Alzheimer's disease. J Geriatr Psychiatry Neurol 2009;22:207–12.

36. Rosenthal MJ, Fajardo M, Gilmore S, et al. Hospitalization and mortality of diabetes in older adults. A 3-year prospective study. Diabetes Care 1998;21:231–5.
37. Morley JE, Flood JF. Psychosocial aspects of diabetes mellitus in older persons. J Am Geriatr Soc 1990;38:605–6.
38. Tariq SH, Tumosa N, Chibnall JT, et al. Comparison of the Saint Louis University mental status examination and the mini-mental state examination for detecting dementia and mild neurocognitive disorder—a pilot study. Am J Geriatr Psychiatry 2006;14:900–10.
39. Banks WA, Morley JE. Memories are made of this: recent advances in understanding cognitive impairments and dementia. J Gerontol A Biol Sci Med Sci 2003;58:314–21.
40. Kaufer DI, Williams CS, Braaten AJ, et al. Cognitive screening for dementia and mild cognitive impairment in assisted living: comparison of 3 tests. J Am Med Dir Assoc 2008;9:586–93.
41. de Tullio MB, Morelli L, Castano EM. The irreversible binding of amyloid peptide substrates to insulin-degrading enzyme: a biological perspective. Prion 2008;2:51–6.
42. Morley JE, Farr SA, Banks WA, et al. A physiological role for amyloid-beta protein: enhancement of learning and memory. J Alzheimers Dis 2009. [Epub ahead of print].
43. Dhamoon MS, Noble JM, Craft S. Intranasal insulin improves cognition and modulates beta-amyloid in early AD. Neurology 2009;72:292–3.
44. Joshi S, Morley JE. Cognitive impairment. Med Clin North Am 2006;90:769–87.
45. Morley JE. Should all long-term care residents receive vitamin D? J Am Med Dir Assoc 2007;8:69–70.
46. Munir J, Wright RJ, Carr DB. A quality improvement study on calcium and vitamin D supplementation in long-term care. J Am Med Dir Assoc 2007;8(2 Suppl 2):e19–23.
47. Drinka PJ, Krause PF, Nest LJ, et al. Determinants of vitamin D levels in nursing home residents. J Am Med Dir Assoc 2007;8:76–9.
48. Hamid Z, Riggs A, Spencer T, et al. Vitamin D deficiency in residents of academic long-term care facilities despite having been prescribed vitamin D. J Am Med Dir Assoc 2007;8:71–5.
49. Perry III HM, Horowitz M, Morley JE, et al. Longitudinal changes in serum 25-hydroxyvitamin D in older people. Metabolism 1999;48:1028–32.
50. Dharmarajan TS. Falls and fractures linked to anemia, delirium osteomalacia, medications, and more: the path to success is strewn with obstacles! J Am Med Dir Assoc 2007;8:549–50.
51. Annweiler C, Allali G, Allain P, et al. Vitamin D and cognitive performance in adults: a systematic review. Eur J Neurol 2009;16:1083–9.
52. Lee DM, Tajar A, Ulubaev A, et al. Association between 25-hydroxyvitamin D levels and cognitive performance in middle-aged and older European men. J Neurol Neurosurg Psychiatr 2009;80:722–9.
53. Buell JS, Scott TM, Dawson-Hughes B, et al. Vitamin D is associated with cognitive function in elders receiving home health services. J Gerontol A Biol Sci Med Sci 2009;64:888–95.
54. Morley JE. Vitamin D redux. J Am Med Dir Assoc 2009;10:591–2.
55. Sultana R, Perluigi M, Butterfield DA. Oxidatively modified proteins in Alzheimer's disease (AD), mild cognitive impairment and animal models of AD: role of Abeta in pathogenesis. Acta Neuropathol 2009;118:131–50.
56. Isaac MG, Quinn R, Tabet N. Vitamin E for Alzheimer's disease and mild cognitive impairment. Cochrane Database Syst Rev 2008;(3):CD002854.

57. Flood JF, Morley JE. Learning and memory in the SAMP8 mouse. Neurosci Biobehav Rev 1998;22:1–20.
58. Petursdottir AL, Farr SA, Morley JE, et al. Lipid perioxidation I brain during aging in the senescence-accelerated mouse (SAM). Neurobiol Aging 2007;28:1170–8.
59. Poon HF, Farr SA, Banks WA, et al. Proteomic identification of less oxidized brain proteins in aged senescence-accelerated mice following administration of anti-sense oligonucleotide directed at the Abeta region of amyloid precursor protein. Brain Res Mol Brain Res 2005;138:8–16.
60. Poon HF, Joshi G, Sultana R, et al. Antisense directed at the Abeta region of APP decreases brain oxidative markers in aged senescence accelerated mice. Brain Res 2004;1018:86–96.
61. Poon HF, Castegna A, Farr SA, et al. Quantitative proteomics analysis of specific protein expression and oxidative modification in aged senescence-accelerated-prone 8 mice brain. Neuroscience 2004;126:915–26.
62. Farr SA, Poon HF, Dognukol-Ak D, et al. The antioxidants alpha-lipoic acid and N-acetylcysteine reverse memory impairment and brain oxidative stress in aged SAMP8 mice. J Neurochem 2003;84:1173–83.
63. Banks WA, Farr SA, La Scola ME, et al. Intravenous human interleukin-1 alpha impairs memory processing in mice: dependence on blood-brain barrier transport into posterior division of the septum. J Pharmacol Exp Ther 2001;299:536–41.
64. Poon HF, Farr SA, Thongboonkerd V, et al. Proteomic analysis of specific brain proteins in aged SAMP8 mice treated with alpha-lipoic acid: implications for aging and age-related neurodegenerative disorders. Neurochem Int 2005;46:159–68.
65. de Freitas RM. Lipoic acid increases hippocampal choline acetyltransferase and acetylcholinersterase activites and improvement memory in epileptic rats. Neurochem Res 2009. [Epub ahead of print].
66. Shenk JC, Liu J, Fischbach K, et al. The effect of acetyl-L-carnitine and R-alpha-lipoic acid treatment in ApoE4 mouse as a model of human Alzheimer's disease. J Neurol Sci 2009;283(1-2):199–206.
67. Suchy J, Chan A, Shea TB. Dietary supplementation with a combination of alpha-lipoic acid, acetyl-L-carnitine, glycerophosphocoline, docosahexaenoic acid, and phosphatidylserine reduces oxidative damage to murine brain and improves cognitive performance. Nutr Res 2009;29:70–4.
68. Moreira PI, Harris PL, Zhu X, et al. Lipoic acid and N-acetyl cysteine decrease mitochondrial-related oxidative stress in Alzheimer disease patient fibroblasts. J Alzheimers Dis 2007;12:195–206.
69. Singh U, Jialal I. Alpha-lipoic acid supplementation and diabetes. Nutr Rev 2008;66:646–57.
70. Packer L, Witt EH, Tritschler HJ. Alpha-Lipoic acid as a biological antioxidant. Free Radic Biol Med 1995;19:227–50.
71. Banks WA, Farr SA, Morley JE. Entry of blood-borne cytokines into the central nervous system: effects on cognitive processes. Neuroimmunomodulation 2002-2003;10:319–27.
72. Haren MT, Malmstrom TK, Miller DK, et al. Higher C-Reactive protein and soluble tumor necrosis factor receptor levels are associated with poor physical function and disability: a cross-sectional analysis of a cohort of late middle-aged African Americans. J Gerontol A Biol Sci Med Sci 2009. [Epub ahead of print].
73. Hager K, Kenklies M, McAfoose J, et al. Alpha-lipoic acid as a new treatment option for Alzheimer's disease—A 48 months follow-up analysis. J Neural Transm Suppl 2007;72:189–93.

74. Sauer J, Tabet N, Howard R. Alpha lipoic acid for dementia. Cochrane Database Syst Rev 2004;(1):CD004244.

75. Féart C, Samieri C, Rondeau V, et al. Adherence to a Mediterranean diet, cognitive decline, and risk of dementia. JAMA 2009;302:638–48.

76. Huang TL, Zandi PP, Tucker KL, et al. Benefits of fatty fish on dementia risk are stronger for those without APOE epsilon4. Neurology 2005;65:1409–14.

77. Dangour AD, Allen E, Elbourne D, et al. Fish consumption and cognitive function among older people in the UK: baseline data from the OPAL study. J Nutr Health Aging 2009;13:198–202.

78. Morris MC. The role of nutrition in Alzheimer's disease: epidemiological evidence. Eur J Neurol 2009;16(Suppl 1):1–7.

79. Petursdottir AL, Farr SA, Morley JE, et al. Effect of dietary n-3 polyunsaturated fatty acids on brain lipid fatty acid composition, learning ability, and memory of senescence-accelerated mouse. J Gerontol A Biol Sci Med Sci 2008;63:1153–60.

80. Kumar VB, Vyas K, Buddhiraju M, et al. Changes in membrane fatty acids and delta-9 desaturase in senescence accelerated (SAMP8) mouse hippocampus with aging. Life Sci 1999;65:1657–62.

81. Cherubini A, Andres-Lacueva C, Martin A, et al. Low plasma N-3 fatty acids and dementia in older persons: the InCHIANTI study. J Gerontol A Biol Sci Med Sci 2007;62:1120–6.

82. Joseph JA, Shukitt-Hale B, Willis LM. Grape juice, berries, and walnuts affect brain aging and behavior. J Nutr 2009;139:1813S–7S.

83. Shukitt-Hale B, Lau FC, Carey AN, et al. Blueberry polyphenols attenuate kainic acid-induced decrements in cognition and alter inflammatory gene expression in rat hippocampus. Nutr Neurosci 2008;11:172–82.

84. Lim GP, Chu T, Yang F, et al. The curry spice curcumin reduces oxidative damage and amyloid pathology in an Alzheimer transgenic mouse. J Neurosci 2001;21:8370–7.

85. Ringman JM, Frautschy SA, Cole GM, et al. A potential role of the curry spice curcumin in Alzheimer's disease. Curr Alzheimer Res 2005;2:131–6.

86. Ng TP, Chiam PC, Lee T, et al. Curry consumption and cognitive function in the elderly. Am J Epidemiol 2006;164:898–906.

87. Knopman DS. Mediterranean diet and late-life cognitive impairment: a taste of benefit. JAMA 2009;302:686–7.

88. Scarmeas N, Stern Y, Mayeux R, et al. Mediterranean diet and mild cognitive impairment. Arch Neurol 2009;66:216–25.

89. Wurtman RJ, Cansev M, Ulus IH. Synapse formation is enhanced by oral administration of uridine and DHA, the circulating precursors of brain phospatides. J Nutr Health Aging 2009;13:189–97.

90. Wurtman RJ, Cansev M, Sakamoto T, et al. Administration of docosahexaenoic acid, uridine and choline increases levels of synaptic membranes and dendritic spines in rodent brain. World Rev Nutr Diet 2009;99:71–96.

91. Holguin S, Huang Y, Liu J, et al. Chronic administration of DHA and UMP improves the impaired memory of environmentally improverished rats. Behav Brain Res 2008;191:11–6.

92. Johnson EJ, McDonald K, Caldarella SM, et al. Cognitive findings of an exploratory trial of docosahexaenoic acid supplementation in older women. Nutr Neurosci 2008;11:75–83.

Healthy Brain Aging: Role of Cognitive Reserve, Cognitive Stimulation, and Cognitive Exercises

Asenath La Rue, PhD

KEYWORDS

- Aging • Cognition • Cognitive stimulation • Training
- Alzheimer disease

The final decade of the 1900s was called the Decade of the Brain, in recognition of advances in science and technology that provided unprecedented views of the human brain in action and enhanced appreciation of the complexity and resilience of the normally functioning brain. The coming decade may well become the Decade of Brain Fitness, as scientists, clinicians, and entrepreneurs test the limits of current knowledge for improving and sustaining human cognitive function to the end of life.

Americans believe that they can improve their brain health through their lifestyle choices. In a recent poll[1] of middle-aged and older adults, 88% endorsed the idea that brain health can be improved (35% said "a little" and 53% said "a lot"). Eighty-four percent reported that they were doing things to improve their brain health, including arts, crafts, hobbies, games and puzzles, and exercising physically.

This article critically examines current knowledge about the role of cognitively stimulating lifestyles and cognitive training interventions in preserving cognitive performance in later life. The emphasis is on optimizing cognitive well-being in normally aging older persons, and, to a lesser extent, on the question of delaying or preventing dementing disorders such as Alzheimer disease (AD). Suggestions for advising patients about brain-healthy lifestyles are provided, cautioned by the recognition that major gaps exist in our knowledge of how best to engineer a cognitively healthy old age.

This work was supported by Grant No. 5R01AG27161 from the National Institute on Aging and the Helen Bader Foundation.
Wisconsin Alzheimer's Institute, School of Medicine and Public Health, University of Wisconsin – Madison, 7818 Big Sky Drive, Suite 215, Madison, WI 53719, USA
E-mail address: larue@wisc.edu

Clin Geriatr Med 26 (2010) 99–111
doi:10.1016/j.cger.2009.11.003
0749-0690/10/$ – see front matter

KEY TERMS, CONCEPTS, AND HYPOTHESES

Terms such as brain health and brain fitness are popular but seldom defined. Paralleling current definitions for physical fitness,[2] brain fitness could be defined as attributes that people have or achieve that relate to the ability to perform cognitive activity. The emphasis in this definition is on function (ie, cognition in action in the everyday world) rather than on brain structure, and, in this regard, it is important to recognize that there are multiple, partially distinct components of cognitive function, including attention, learning and memory, language, visuospatial processing, reasoning, and executive skills. Individuals may be fit in terms of language and communication, but less fit in memory or attention, and different interventions may be needed to improve fitness in each area. Optimal brain fitness requires the absence of brain disease or systemic illness that critically affects the brain, but persons with brain injury, or those experiencing early stages of a degenerative brain disease, may be more or less fit depending on their genetic predispositions, endowments garnered from early life experiences, and current lifestyle choices.

Concepts such as brain reserve and cognitive reserve have gained prominence in discussions of the differential attributes that individuals have for coping with the challenges of brain injury or brain disease. Brain reserve generally refers to the structural neural substrate (eg, brain size or neuronal count) that supports cognitive function. Given the same degree of AD brain pathology, for example, individuals with larger brains are less likely to exhibit clinical symptoms of dementia than those with smaller brains.[3] Similarly, healthy older adults with high executive function have increased cortical thickness in certain key brain regions compared with those with average executive function.[4] Cognitive reserve refers to the brain's capacity to actively cope with brain damage through the implementation of cognitive processes. Two individuals with the same degree of structural brain reserve might adapt to brain injury more or less successfully if one has more cognitive reserve, that is, more cognitive processes to enlist or to use in compensation. Epidemiologic studies have shown that the risk of AD is lower for persons with higher levels of education, higher occupational attainment, or higher premorbid intelligence quotient (IQ),[5,6] and, because of such observations, education and occupation are often used as proxies in predicting who is likely to have more or less cognitive reserve. Functional neuroimaging studies have begun to document associations relevant to cognitive reserve.[5] For example, in one recent study,[7] cognitively healthy older adults with higher cognitive reserve (as estimated by IQ, education/occupation, and activities), had larger magnetic resonance imaging (MRI)-derived whole brain volumes and reduced brain activity during cognitive processing, presumably because they were making more efficient use of cognitive networks. In patients with mild AD, by contrast, those with higher cognitive reserve had smaller brain volumes, but increased brain activity, suggesting active attempts at cognitive compensation, despite more advanced neuropathology. **Fig. 1** shows how cognitive reserve might mediate between AD pathology and its clinical expression. The concepts of brain reserve and cognitive reserve may be relevant to understanding individual differences in coping with a wide range of dementing disorders (eg, frontotemporal dementia[8]; dementia with Lewy bodies).[9]

There is increasing recognition that the neuropathologic substrates of AD begin years or even decades before clinical diagnosis,[10] raising the possibility of intervening at preclinical stages to prevent the disease, or at least delay the onset of clinically significant symptoms. At present, there are no known treatments or lifestyle modifications that can prevent the progression of AD pathology. However, the hypothesis that onset of clinical symptoms may be delayed by interventions is attracting great

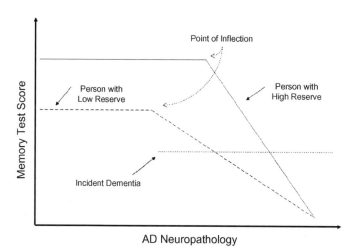

Fig. 1. Theoretic illustration of how cognitive reserve may mediate between AD pathology and its clinical expression. Note that for a person with high cognitive reserve, it is hypothesized that the point of inflection at which memory begins to be affected by AD pathology is later than for a person with low cognitive reserve, and that at any level of memory performance, AD pathology is more severe for the person with high cognitive reserve. Once clinical dementia begins, however, clinical progression is hypothesized to advance more rapidly for the person with high cognitive reserve. (*From* Stern Y. Cognitive reserve. Neuropsychologia 2009;47:2017; with permission.)

attention, and several prospective studies are underway to identify risk and protective factors and to pinpoint when in the lifespan each factor may have the most pronounced impact on AD pathology and symptom progression. This view of AD, as one among many chronic diseases that are not currently curable, but may be preventable to some degree, reflects an important shift in mindset among researchers and clinicians in the field. This view is referred to in this article as the prevention hypothesis, although it might be more realistic to call it the forestalling hypothesis. **Fig. 2** shows hypothetical impacts of earlier interventions on slowing the rate of cognitive decline. By the time clinical dementia emerges, affected individuals have already experienced extensive brain impairment, lessening the odds that cognitive symptoms can be effectively ameliorated. The same may be true of mild cognitive impairment (MCI), which is often a precursor of AD.

COGNITIVELY STIMULATING LIFESTYLES: WHAT IS KNOWN?

Most epidemiologic studies that have examined cognitive stimulation as a lifestyle variable have found slower rates of cognitive decline among those who routinely engage in more cognitively demanding tasks compared with those with a more mentally sedentary lifestyles.[6,11] Many of these same studies have also shown a reduced risk for AD and other dementias among more cognitively active persons.

One recent population-based study[12] of cognitively healthy adults 65 years and older found that a 1-point increase in frequency of engagement across 7 cognitive activities (reading books; reading magazines; reading newspapers; playing cards, checkers, crosswords, or other puzzles; going to a museum; viewing television; and listening to the radio) was associated with a 64% reduction in odds of developing

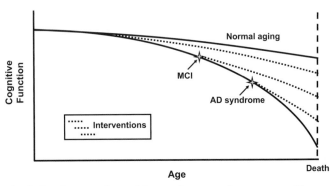

Fig. 2. Hypothetical trajectory of cognitive performance for persons with normally aging brains, MCI and AD. If interventions can be identified to slow the course of AD pathology or symptom expression, intervening before MCI or AD is diagnosed is likely to have the greatest beneficial impact. (*Courtesy of* Mark A. Sager, MD, Madison, WI.)

dementia over a 4-year period; on average, individuals with cognitive activity scores at the 10th percentile were twice as likely to develop dementia as those with cognitive activity scores at the 90th percentile. On the scale used by Wilson and colleagues, a 1-point increase in the cognitive activity scale would correspond, for example, to engaging in a cognitive activity daily rather than several times per week, or several times a week rather than several times a month. The most pronounced difference in AD risk was between cognitively inactive lifestyles compared with an average level of cognitive activity, with smaller additional benefit seen from the average to highly active range.

Another prospective study of nondemented persons 75 years and older[13] found that those in the highest one-third of cognitive activity (corresponding to 11 activity days per week from a set of 6 activities consisting of reading books or newspapers, writing for pleasure, doing crossword puzzles, playing board games or cards, participating in organized group discussions, and playing musical instruments) had a 63% lower risk of developing dementia in the next 5 years than those in the lowest third of cognitive activity. Reading, playing board games, and playing musical instruments were the activities most closely linked to dementia odds.

Although each of these investigations came to similar conclusions regarding the potentially protective role of cognitively stimulating lifestyles, the specific activities that they found to be beneficial varied. An earlier epidemiologic study conducted in France reported lower AD risk with traveling, doing odd jobs, knitting, and gardening.[14] None of the epidemiologic studies of leisure-time cognitive activities have attempted to validate engagement through direct observation or informant report, and most do not assess duration or intensity of engagement in cognitively stimulating activities. The overall conclusion from these observational studies is encouraging and lends some support to the general idea that "more is better" when it comes to cognitive stimulation, but it is clear that the field lacks a metric (ie, a cognitive yardstick) for measuring the types or amount of activities that would be most beneficial.

Questions of cause and effect are unanswered in this area of research.[15] Is lowered engagement in cognitive leisure activities before the onset of dementia due to prodromal disease that makes the performance of these activities more difficult and less appealing? Is engagement in cognitively demanding leisure activities simply a marker for generally higher intellectual ability or a byproduct of higher education? A few studies have used statistical modeling and long-term follow-up to try to shed light on these questions. Schooler and Mulato[16] followed a representative sample of more than 600 employed men (average age = 64 years at baseline) and their spouses over a period of 20 years. The focus of their study was on the preservation of intellectual flexibility in relation to the cognitive complexity of leisure activities. Across this lengthy follow-up, they found evidence for reciprocal (ie, bidirectional) associations; that is, initial high levels of intellectual functioning led to high levels of cognitive complexity in activities, which, in turn, resulted in higher levels of intellectual functioning. These researchers concluded that: "...our findings strongly suggest that...doing substantively complex tasks...is an 'analog of aerobic exercise,'" but, again, these conclusions are based on observational research. Studies relating work histories to cognitive preservation are relevant to Schooler's substantive complexity hypothesis.[17] Individuals whose main occupations require engagement with data or people in complex ways are more likely to maintain cognitive skills as they age[17,18] than those with less intellectually or socially demanding jobs. Retirement may reduce some of the cognitive benefits of stimulating work, at least in the short term.[19]

Crowe and colleagues,[20] reporting on a long-term follow-up of twin pairs discordant for development of AD, found that higher levels of intellectual-cultural activities in middle age were associated with reduced risk of AD 20 years later. Similar associations have been reported between cognitively complex work in middle age and dementia risk in late life.[21] With such lengthy follow-up intervals, the possibility that cognitively inactive lifestyles might be due to prodromal dementia becomes less plausible, but other possible confounds cannot be ruled out.

Older adults with higher levels of education or higher estimated IQ tend to engage more often in cognitively demanding leisure activities than persons with lesser education or lower IQ. It is not clear yet whether individuals' choices of leisure activities influence cognitive trajectories more than what might be expected based on their education and general ability level. Several studies suggest at least partially independent effects of these different factors,[22,23] and at least one major epidemiologic study found that frequency of recent cognitive leisure activity had a stronger link to AD risk than education or occupational level.[24]

Lifestyles that combine cognitively stimulating activities with physical activities and rich social networks may provide the best odds of preserving cognitive function in old age. In a 9-year follow-up of a healthy aging sample in Sweden, individuals who were active on any of these key dimensions (cognitive, physical, and social) had lowered dementia risk, but those who were active on 2 or all 3 dimensions had the lowest risk of all.[25]

COGNITIVE TRAINING INTERVENTIONS: WHAT IS KNOWN?

It is well documented that older adults benefit from direct training programs that focus on specific cognitive skills. A meta-analytical review of memory training concluded that there are reliable gains in memory performance from participation in memory training classes, and that the effect is robust (average gain with training = 0.73 SD vs 0.38 SD for controls) across many different studies and samples.[26,27] However, several important questions have been raised about this research. Many early studies were based on small and select samples, and, in some cases, benefits were short-lived once training was discontinued. More recent studies continue to report positive outcomes from training specific cognitive skills, but the strength and significance of training effects are open to differing interpretations (for contrasting reviews, see Refs.[28,29]).

The Advanced Cognitive Training for Independent and Vital Elderly (ACTIVE) study was the first large-scale randomized controlled trial of the effects of cognitive training for nondemented older adults.[30] The sample consisted of 2832 community-residing volunteers aged 65 to 94 years (mean = 73 years) recruited from 6 sites across the United States. All had Mini Mental State Examination (MMSE) scores of 23 or higher and were free of significant functional deficits at the start of the study. The design was randomized, single blind with 4 groups: memory training, reasoning training, speed-of-processing training, and no-contact control. Participants were trained in small groups for 10 1-hour sessions over a 5 to 6 week period. Each training program produced an immediate positive effect on its corresponding cognitive ability (as measured on similar tasks). Gains were especially noticeable for speed-of-processing and reasoning training, with a more modest benefit from memory training. Subsequent follow-ups have shown that modest benefits persist from training for at least 5 years.[31] The ACTIVE study provides good evidence that even a small amount of training can benefit specific cognitive skills and that the benefits persist to some degree for extended periods of time. An important limitation in outcomes, however, is that training benefits were task-specific and usually did not extend to apparently similar, more naturalistic cognitive tasks (eg, remembering a shopping list rather than a list of unrelated words of the type used in training). Despite this, at 5 years post training, participants in the ACTIVE training program were less likely than controls to have declines in health-related quality of life,[32] suggesting that well-designed cognitive training interventions could have benefits for important aspects of everyday life.

Cognitive researchers have begun to explore other types of training programs in the hope of finding more generalized benefits. One commercially available program, Brain Fitness, marketed by Posit Science, consists of an online program of graduated cognitive exercises designed to enhance brain plasticity.[33] In the largest outcome study to date,[34] 487 cognitively healthy and well-educated older adults (mean age = 75 years) were randomly assigned to experimental training with the Brain Fitness program or an active control condition where they spent an equivalent number of hours on content-oriented coursework. The experimental program emphasized procedural learning (ie, learning "how" rather than "what") that involved practice with auditory language processing (tracking and comparing sounds of increasing complexity) for 60 minutes per day, 5 days per week for 8 to 10 weeks. Testing at the end of training indicated large benefits on auditory processing speed, moderate benefits on self-reported everyday cognitive skills, and small but statistically significant benefits on memory performance. In this study, too, training primarily benefited skills most closely related to those used in training, but there was some evidence for more generalized benefits. Other studies with the Brain Fitness program have shown that benefits persist to some degree for at least 3 months,[35] but longer-term results are not available.

Could standard, commercial video games help to sustain older adults' cognitive skills? There is some preliminary positive evidence. In a recent small-scale study,[36] 40 cognitively healthy older adults were randomly assigned to a video game practice group or a no-contact control group. The experimental group engaged in approximately 24 hours of practice with a strategy-based real-time video game over a 7- to 8-week period. Participants improved their speed of completion and game scores over time, but, more importantly, scores on unrelated, standardized tests of executive function also improved for the experimental group relative to controls. The investigators speculated that the greater transfer of training observed with the video game practice may have been due to the constantly shifting task priorities necessitated by these games, which required flexibility and rapid response. It is not known yet how long benefits from playing such games might persist or whether skills besides executive function might be enhanced.

In their review of recent training studies, Green and Bavelier[37] conclude that lasting, generalized cognitive benefits are unlikely to come from brain-training regimes that focus on one type of task, and that more durable, generalized benefits may come from tasks that are complex and tap many systems in parallel. If this is the case, natural training regimes (eg, video games) may prove more beneficial for sustaining older adults' cognition than current programs that have been specifically designed for the purpose of brain training. Other novel training approaches designed to increase the breadth and persistence of training benefits (for a review, see Ref.[38]) include collaborative training models, in which older adults engage in cooperative problem solving[39]; wellness programs that combine cognitive training with physical exercise[40]; and programs designed to enhance cognitive skills through engagement in volunteer activities such as literacy training with children.[41]

Will any cognitive training program prove useful in delaying the onset of clinical dementia? There are no data available on this question. The obstacles to a clinical trial that could address this question are significant. Long-term follow-up would be needed, and it is likely that only a sustained and varied training program could hope to produce this important benefit. In the literature at present, the paucity of follow-up results, small sample sizes, and heterogeneous methods of training and measuring outcomes suggest that caution is needed in promoting the potential of structured cognitive interventions for healthy older adults.[28]

Cognitive training can produce modest, specific benefits for persons with preclinical cognitive conditions such as MCI or with varying degrees of dementia. Belleville and colleagues[42] observed strong gains in face-name memory for a small group of MCI patients given practice and memory-strategy training compared with a no-intervention control. By contrast, the ACTIVE study reported that participants who had lower memory scores but no dementia at baseline (possible MCI cases) benefited significantly from reasoning and speed-of-processing training, but not from memory training.[43] There have also been several case examples and small-sample studies illustrating that specialized interventions such as spaced-retrieval training can improve recall of names and other practical skills among patients with AD,[44,45] and improvement on standard memory measures has been reported from a program that combined computerized attention and sensory processing activities with pencil-and-paper exercises such as mazes, crossword puzzles, and anagrams in a small group of persons with mild to moderate dementia.[46] However, larger-scale trials of these types of interventions are needed in persons with MCI and AD to establish clinical efficacy.[47] Research to date has been limited by lack of adequate controls, small sample sizes, and interventions that combine multiple training techniques and approaches, making it difficult to assess the contributions of any individual strategy.[48]

POTENTIAL MECHANISMS FOR NEUROPROTECTIVE EFFECTS OF COGNITIVE STIMULATION AND TRAINING

The mechanisms by which cognitively stimulating activities might promote brain and cognitive reserve are unknown, but multiple modes of effect have been hypothesized.

A growing number of animal studies suggest that cognitive stimulation may have direct effects on the brain substrates that support cognition. Stimulating environments and physical exercise promote neurogenesis in the dentate gyrus in mice[49] and increase neuronal plasticity and resistance to cell death.[50] Exposure to such environments may also slow or prevent accumulation of key indictors of AD pathology, β-amyloid levels and amyloid pathology, in transgenic mice.[51] It is not known yet how extensively similar brain changes occur in response to cognitively stimulating environments in humans, or whether processes such as hippocampal neurogenesis are causally related to preserved brain function.[50] In a recent human study focusing on physical exercise,[52] an aerobic exercise program was found to increase cerebral blood flow in the dentate gyrus, and blood flow, in turn, correlated with performance on a memory task, suggesting to the researchers that dentate gyrus cerebral blood flow may provide an imaging correlate of exercise-induced neurogenesis. This same technique might be valuable in studying effects of cognitive training programs. A host of mechanisms for brain plasticity and compensation other than neurogenesis are being investigated, including dendritic length and branching, synaptic modulations, neuronal morphology, neural network redundancies, and neurochemical effects.[53–57]

Functional neuroimaging studies are being used to identify brain regions and cognitive processes that mediate cognitive reserve.[5] Much of the work to date has focused on understanding the brain regions involved in performance of specific memory tasks and on whether there are age differences in the extent or pattern of brain activation during task performance. Two major findings have emerged. On some tasks, young and old persons activate the same or similar brain regions; as task difficulty increases, the magnitude of activation is often higher among older individuals, suggesting that greater effort is required among the old to achieve a comparable level of performance. On other tasks, older subjects sometimes recruit (ie, activate) additional brain regions, not used by the young, while performing a memory task. The first finding may be an example of age-related differences in neural network efficiency, whereas the latter may be an example of active neural compensation. Heightened activation or recruitment of additional brain regions sometimes correlates with estimates of brain reserve (eg, IQ or years of education), and sometimes not, and the pattern of correlations can differ for younger and older adults.

Recently, neuroimaging researchers have begun to search for substrates of a more general cognitive reserve network that might support performance across a broader range of tasks. It is this type of reserve that could provide the basis for sustaining everyday cognitive performance in the face of advancing brain change due to age or incipient AD. Only preliminary results are available. Stern and colleagues[58] identified a network of brain regions in younger adults that was activated during performance on two different memory tasks and was positively correlated with estimates of cognitive reserve. The activated regions (bilateral superior frontal gyrus, bilateral medial frontal gyrus, and left middle frontal gyrus) support cognitive control processes (eg, working memory or attentional switching), suggesting that individuals with greater cognitive reserve may have generally enhanced control over their cognitive processing. In this study, however, the pattern of brain activation was less consistent across tasks for older subjects, so the role of a more general cognitive reserve network is unclear at this point.

IMPLICATIONS FOR CLINICAL PRACTICE AND PUBLIC HEALTH POLICY

There is a great deal of evidence that older adults retain the ability to learn new things, and observational studies show that cognitively active older persons are more likely to retain their cognitive abilities than those who are cognitively inactive. What is not known is whether a cognitively active lifestyle, or participation in specific cognitive training programs, can prevent or delay the onset of clinical dementia. Given limitations in current knowledge, it can be difficult to answer patients' questions about the best things to do to increase the odds of healthy cognitive aging. However, the risks of harm from recommending a cognitively active lifestyle, or enrollment in a memory training class, are small.

Table 1 lists recommendations that the author currently uses in discussions with clients who are interested in mental activities that might promote brain fitness. As the literature on mental exercise and cognition grows, more specific recommendations may become possible.

The possibility of improving and sustaining brain fitness is beginning to affect public policy. In 2007, the Centers for Disease Control and Prevention issued a *National Public Health Road Map to Maintaining Cognitive Health* in partnership with the Alzheimer's Association, the American Association of Retired Persons, the Administration on Aging, and others.[59] The emphasis is on preserving cognitive function, rather than on preventing dementia, and the goals are largely aspirational (eg, to "help people understand the connection between risk and protective factors and cognitive health"). The emphasis on primary prevention for large and diverse communities is ambitious, and it may set in motion a natural experiment, which, over time, may inform us of the success and limitations of a public-health approach.

Funding is needed to study potential benefits of nonpharmacologic interventions on brain fitness, including cognitive stimulation and training. Only a small fraction of federal dollars for research are devoted to interventions other than drugs, and private funds are hard to attract outside of the commercial product realm. If this continues, many more products for brain health are likely to be marketed, including more brain games, with little or no evidence of efficacy.

Table 1
Recommendations for a cognitively active lifestyle

Recommendation	Rationale
Make time for cognitively stimulating activities that you've always enjoyed	Continuing favorite activities can ensure sustainability of cognitive stimulation. Long-term exposure to cognitive stimulation may be needed for practical functional benefits
Add some new cognitive challenges, as your time and enjoyment permit	Trying new activities may enhance brain plasticity by requiring new learning or development of new cognitive strategies
Aim to engage in cognitively stimulating activities several times a week or more...generate some mental sweat	Current knowledge does not permit a prescription for how often or how long individuals should engage in cognitively stimulating activities. However, epidemiologic studies suggest that more is better, within clinically reasonable limits
Be aware that there is no 1 cognitive activity, or combination of activities, that is uniquely good for reducing AD risk	Many different types of cognitively stimulating activities have been associated with preserved cognitive skill. There are no data yet to show that cognitive activities prevent or delay AD
Social interactions can be a great way to stimulate the mind	Group training of cognitive skills has been shown to be effective in sharpening specific cognitive skills, and broader social networks have been associated with reduced AD risk

KEY GAPS IN RESEARCH AND SUGGESTIONS ON HOW TO FILL THESE GAPS

To better understand the roles of cognitive stimulation and cognitive training in sustaining cognitive function in healthy older people, and in possibly preventing or delaying the onset of AD, conceptual and methodological advances are needed, in addition to more research.

A few of the key gaps in research, and suggestions for addressing these gaps, are outlined below.

- There is currently no metric for measuring cognitive stimulation or comparing the relative stimulating properties of different cognitive activities. Each study in this area has measured cognitive activity in unique ways, and in most cases, little effort has been made to establish the reliability and validity of cognitive activity measures. In contrast to the realm of physical activity, in which classification systems have been developed that permit the comparison of total energy expenditure across diverse physical tasks, there is no such common metric for cognitive stimulation or cognitive effort. At a minimum, it would be helpful for researchers who are studying cognitive leisure activities to adopt a standard tool for measuring these activities, to fast-track the development of more specific guidelines regarding the intensity, duration, and types of activities that are most beneficial.
- Concepts such as brain reserve and cognitive reserve are heuristically useful, but, as currently used, they do not explain how increased coping comes about. More basic research is needed to increase understanding of how factors such as higher initial education, or more cognitively stimulating leisure activities, may be affecting the brain, structurally and functionally.
- The practical effect of cognitive training programs remains to be demonstrated. Although cognitive training clearly benefits specifically trained skills, more research is needed to address questions of practical importance and to design training programs which cross-train multiple skills of the types that might enhance transfer of training to everyday situations. More randomized controlled trials of the type used in ACTIVE are needed, using broader and more ambitious training regimes. Programs that promote activities and lifestyles that embody what Schooler calls *substantive complexity*[16,60] warrant further study.[39]
- There is no evidence yet that cognitively stimulating activities or cognitive training programs delay or prevent dementia. Longer-term follow-up studies are needed to assess whether or not participation in cognitive training programs or adoption of cognitively stimulating lifestyles forestalls the expression of clinical dementia or affects neurobiology in disease-modifying ways. There is also a need to learn when in the lifespan such experiences would be most beneficial. Environmental stimulation and education in childhood and youth are probably critical in setting the stage for brain reserve, but, from a public health perspective, there is also a need to know whether choices made in midlife and later can reliably sustain or add to cognitive reserve.

REFERENCES

1. American Society on Aging and Metlife Foundation. Attitudes and awareness of brain health poll, 2006. Available at: http://www.asaging.org/asav2/mindalert/pdfs/BH.pdf. Accessed September 29, 2009.
2. US Department of Health and Human Services. Healthy people 2010. 2nd edition. Washington, DC: US Government Printing Office; 2000. Available

at: http://www.healthypeople.gov/Document/HTML/Volume2/22Physical.htm. Accessed September 29, 2009.

3. Katzman R, Terry T, DeTeresa R, et al. Clinical, pathological, and neurochemical changes in dementia: a subgroup with preserved mental status and numerous neocortical plaques. Ann Neurol 1988;23:138–44.

4. Fjell AM, Walhovd KB, Rienvang I, et al. Selective increase of cortical thickness in high-performing elderly – structural indices of optimal cognitive aging. Neuroimage 2006;29:984–94.

5. Stern Y. Cognitive reserve. Neuropsychologia 2009;47:2015–28.

6. Valenzuela MJ, Sachdev P. Brain reserve and dementia: a systematic review. Psychol Med 2005;35:1–14.

7. Solé-Padullés C, Bartrés-Faz D, Junqué C, et al. Brain structure and function related to cognitive reserve variables in normal aging, mild cognitive impairment and Alzheimer's disease. Neurobiol Aging 2009;30:1114–24.

8. Borroni B, Premi E, Agosti C, et al. Revisiting brain reserve hypothesis in frontotemporal dementia: evidence from a brain perfusion study. Dement Geriatr Cogn Disord 2009;28:130–5.

9. Perneckzky R, Drzezga A, Boecker H, et al. FDG PET correlates of impaired activities of daily living in dementia with Lewy bodies: implications for cognitive reserve. Am J Geriatr Psychiatry 2009;17:188–95.

10. Braak H, Braak E. Alzheimer's disease: striatal amyloid deposits and neurofibrillary changes. J Neuropathol Exp Neurol 1990;49:215–24.

11. Fratiglioni L, Paillard-Borg S, Winblad B. An active and socially integrated lifestyle in late life might protect against dementia. Lancet Neurol 2004;3:242–53.

12. Wilson RS, Bennett DA, Bienias JL, et al. Cognitive activity and incident AD in a population-based sample of older persons. Neurology 2002;59:1910–4.

13. Verghese J, Lipton RB, Katz MJ, et al. Leisure activities and the risk of dementia in the elderly. N Engl J Med 2003;348:2508–16.

14. Fabrigoule C, Letenneur L, Dartingues JF, et al. Social and leisure activities and risk of dementia: a prospective longitudinal study. J Am Geriatr Soc 1995;43:485–90.

15. Salthouse TA. Mental exercise and mental aging: evaluating the validity of the "use it or lose it" hypothesis. Perspect Psychol Sci 2006;1:68–87.

16. Schooler C, Mulato MS. The reciprocal effects of leisure time activities and intellectual functioning in older people: a longitudinal analysis. Psychol Aging 2001; 16:466–82.

17. Kohn ML, Schooler C. The reciprocal effects of the substantive complexity of work and intellectual flexibility: a longitudinal assessment. Am J Sociol 1978;84: 24–52.

18. Andel R, Kareholt L, Parker M, et al. Complexity of main lifetime occupation and cognition in advanced old age. J Aging Health 2007;19:397–415.

19. Finkel D, Andel R, Gatz M, et al. The role of occupational complexity in trajectories of cognitive aging before and after retirement. Psychol Aging 2009;24: 563–73.

20. Crowe M, Andel R, Pedersen NI, et al. Does participation in leisure activities lead to reduced risk of Alzheimer's disease? A prospective study of Swedish twins. J Gerontol B Psychol Sci Soc Sci 2003;58:P249–55.

21. Karp A, Andel R, Parker MG, et al. Mentally stimulating activities at work during midlife and dementia risk after age 75: follow-up study from the Kungsholmen project. Am J Geriatr Psychiatry 2009;17:227–36.

22. McDowell I, Xi G, Lindsay J, et al. Mapping the connections between education and dementia. J Clin Exp Neuropsychol 2007;29:127–41.

23. Ngandu T, von Strauss E, Helkala E-L, et al. Education and dementia: what lies behind the association. Neurology 2007;69:1442–50.
24. Wilson RS, Bennett DA. Cognitive activity and risk of Alzheimer's disease. Curr Dir Psychol Sci 2003;12:87–91.
25. Karp A, Paillard-Borg S, Wang HX, et al. Mental, physical and social components in leisure activities equally contribute to decrease dementia risk. Dement Geriatr Cogn Disord 2006;21:65–73.
26. Verhaeghen P, Marcoen A, Goosens L. Improving memory performance in the aged through mnemonic training: a meta-analytic study. Psychol Aging 1992;7: 242–51.
27. Neely AS. Multifactorial memory training in normal aging: in search of memory improvement beyond the ordinary. In: Hill RD, Backman L, Neely AS, editors. Cognitive rehabilitation in old age. New York: Oxford University Press; 2000. p. 63–80.
28. Papp KV, Walsh SJ, Snyder PJ. Immediate and delayed effects of cognitive interventions in healthy elderly: a review of current literature and future directions. Alzheimers Dement 2009;5:50–60.
29. Valenzuela M, Sachdev P. Can cognitive exercise prevent the onset of dementia? Systematic review of randomized clinical trials with longitudinal follow-up. Am J Geriatr Psychiatry 2009;17:179–87.
30. Ball K, Berch DB, Heimers KF, et al. Effects of cognitive training interventions with older adults: a randomized controlled trial. JAMA 2002;288:2271–81.
31. Willis SL, Tennstedt SL, Marsiske M, et al. Long-term effects of cognitive training on everyday functional outcomes in older adults. JAMA 2006;296: 2805–14.
32. Wolinsky FD, Unverzagt FW, Smith DM, et al. The ACTIVE training trial and health-related quality of life: protection that lasts 5 years. J Gerontol A Biol Sci Med Sci 2006;61:1324–9.
33. Mahncke HW, Bronstone A, Merzenich MM. Brain plasticity and functional losses in the aged: scientific bases for a novel intervention. Prog Brain Res 2006;157: 81–109.
34. Smith GE, Housen P, Yaffe K, et al. A cognitive training program based on principles of brain plasticity: results from the Improvement in Memory with Plasticity-based Adaptive Cognitive Training (IMPACT) study. J Am Geriatr Soc 2009;57: 594–603.
35. Mahncke HW, Connor BB, Appelman J, et al. Memory enhancement in healthy older adults using a brain plasticity-based training program: a randomized, controlled study. Proc Natl Acad Sci U S A 2006;103:12523–8.
36. Basak C, Boot WR, Voss MW, et al. Can training in a real-time strategy video game attenuate cognitive decline in older adults? Psychol Aging 2008;23: 765–77.
37. Green CS, Bavelier D. Exercising your brain: a review of human brain plasticity and training-induced learning. Psychol Aging 2008;23:692–701.
38. Rebok GW, Carlson MC, Langbaum JBS. Training and maintaining memory abilities in healthy older adults: traditional and novel approaches. J Gerontol B Psychol Sci Soc Sci 2007;62(Spec No 1):53–61.
39. Stine-Morrow EAL, Parisi JM, Morrow DG, et al. The effects of an engaged lifestyle on cognitive vitality: a field experiment. Psychol Aging 2008;23:778–86.
40. Oswald W, Gunzelmann T, Rupprecht R, et al. Differential effects of single versus combined cognitive and physical training with older adults: the SimA study in a 5-year perspective. Eur J Ageing 2006;3:179–92.

41. Carlson MC, Erickson KI, Kramer AF, et al. Evidence for neurocognitive plasticity in at-risk older adults: the experience corps program. J Gerontol A Biol Sci Med Sci 2009;64(12):1275–82.
42. Belleville S, Gilbert B, Fontaine F, et al. Improvement of episodic memory in persons with mild cognitive impairment and healthy older adults: evidence from a cognitive intervention program. Dement Geriatr Cogn Disord 2006;22:486–99.
43. Unverzagt FW, Kasten L, Johnson KE, et al. Effect of memory impairment on training outcomes in ACTIVE. J Int Neuropsychol Soc 2007;13:953–60.
44. Camp CC, Bird MJ, Cherry KE. Retrieval strategies as a rehabilitation aid for cognitive loss in pathological aging. In: Hill RD, Backman L, Neely AS, editors. Cognitive rehabilitation in old age. New York: Oxford University Press; 2000. p. 224–48.
45. Clare L, Wilson BA, Carter G, et al. Relearning face-name associations in early Alzheimer's disease. Neuropsychology 2002;16:538–47.
46. Eckroth-Bucher M, Siberski J. Preserving cognition through an integrated cognitive stimulation and training program. Am J Alzheimers Dis Other Demen 2009; 24:234–45.
47. Clare L, Woods RT, Moniz Cook ED, et al. Cognitive rehabilitation and cognitive training for early-stage Alzheimer's disease and vascular dementia. Cochrane Database Syst Rev 2003;(4):CD003260.
48. Sitzer DI, Twamley EW, Jeste DV. Cognitive training in Alzheimer's disease: a meta-analysis of the literature. Acta Psychiatr Scand 2006;114:75–90.
49. van Praag H, Shubert T, Zhao C, et al. Exercise enhances learning and hippocampal neurogenesis in aged mice. J Neurosci 2005;25:8680–5.
50. Jessberger S, Gage FH. Stem-cell-associated structural and functional plasticity in the aging hippocampus. Psychol Aging 2008;23:684–91.
51. Lazarov O, Robinson J, Tang YP, et al. Environmental enrichment reduces Abeta levels and amyloid deposition in transgenic mice. Cell 2005;120:701–13.
52. Pereira AC, Huddleston DE, Brickman AM, et al. An *in vivo* correlate of exercise-induced neurogenesis in the adult dentate gyrus. Proc Natl Acad Sci U S A 2007; 104:5638–43.
53. Bruckner RL. Memory and executive function in aging and AD: multiple factors that cause decline and reserve factors that compensate. Neuron 2004;44: 195–206.
54. Dauffau H. Brain plasticity: from pathophysiological mechanisms to therapeutic applications. J Clin Neurosci 2006;13:885–97.
55. Savioz A, Leuba G, Vallet PG, et al. Contribution of neural networks to Alzheimer disease's progression. Brain Res Bull 2009;80:309–14.
56. Iacono D, Markesbery WR, Gross M, et al. The nun study: clinically silent AD, neuronal hypertrophy, and linguistic skills in early life. Neurology 2009;73: 665–73.
57. Sachdev PS, Valenzuela M. Brain and cognitive reserve. Am J Geriatr Psychiatry 2009;17:175–8.
58. Stern Y, Zarahn E, Habeck C, et al. A common neural network for cognitive reserve in verbal and object working memory in young but not old. Cereb Cortex 2007;18:959–67.
59. Centers for Disease Control and Prevention and the Alzheimer's Association. The healthy brain initiative: a national public health road map to maintaining cognitive health. Chicago: Alzheimer's Association; 2007.
60. Schooler C. Use it–and keep it, longer, probably. Perspect Psychol Sci 2007;2: 24–9.

Dementia Risk Prediction: Are We There Yet?

Sanjeev M. Kamat, MD[a,b,c,d,*], Anjali S. Kamat, MD[e],
George T. Grossberg, MD[d]

KEYWORDS

- Dementia • Risk factors • Prediction
- Geriatric • Protective factors

Dementia is a term for memory impairment and loss of other intellectual abilities severe enough to cause interference with daily life. Alzheimer disease accounts for 50% to 70% of dementia cases. Other types of dementia include Lewy body dementia, vascular dementia, mixed dementia, and frontotemporal dementia. The precise cause of many dementias, including Alzheimer disease, is not known, but several risk factors that increase the risk for the development of dementia and several protective factors that may protect against the development of dementia are known. As more is understood about the relative importance of individual risk and protective factors, a dementia risk index (DRI) may be able to be developed in the future. Controlling modifiable risk and protective factors is advisable not only in patients with dementia but also in their at-risk family members.

This article reviews potential risk factors and protective factors for the development of dementia, and in particular, Alzheimer disease (AD) and discusses the challenges in developing a DRI.

RISK FACTORS

Age

Increasing age is a risk factor for AD, and the incidence and prevalence rates for AD double every 5 years after the age of 65 years.[1] Currently, around 5.1 million people aged 65 years and older and 200,000 individuals younger than 65 years have AD.[2] It

---

[a] Department of Psychiatry, St Alexius Hospital, 3933 South Broadway, St Louis, MO 63118, USA
[b] Department of Psychiatry, Forest Park Hospital, 6150 Oakland Avenue, St Louis, MO 63139, USA
[c] Department of Psychiatry, Jefferson Regional Medical Center, Highway 61 South, Crystal City, MO 63019, USA
[d] Department of Neurology and Psychiatry, Saint Louis University School of Medicine, 1438 South Grand Boulevard, St Louis, MO 63104, USA
[e] Division of Geriatric Medicine, Department of Internal Medicine, Saint Louis University School of Medicine, 1402 South Grand Boulevard, M238, St Louis, MO 63104, USA
* Corresponding author. Department of Psychiatry, St Alexius Hospital, 3933 South Broadway, St Louis, MO 63118.
E-mail address: kamatsm@gmail.com (S.M. Kamat).

Clin Geriatr Med 26 (2010) 113–123
doi:10.1016/j.cger.2009.12.001   **geriatric.theclinics.com**
0749-0690/10/$ – see front matter © 2010 Elsevier Inc. All rights reserved.

is estimated that as many as 45% of people aged 85 years and older have significant cognitive impairment and dementia.[3]

Sex

As compared with men, women are at a higher risk for developing AD.[4] A pooled analysis of 4 population-based prospective cohort studies was performed, and significant gender differences in the incidence of AD after age 85 years was found. No gender differences in rates or risks for vascular dementia were found.[5] When compared with men, the cumulative risk for a 65-year-old woman to develop AD at the age of 95 years was higher. A recent study by Cankurtaran and colleagues[6] of 203 patients with AD showed that female sex, advanced age, depression, and intake of vitamin supplements were independent related risk factors for AD. Possible reasons for women being at greater risk for developing AD compared with men include longer life span of women (therefore a higher probability of developing dementia) and the loss of the neuroprotective effects of estrogen.[7]

Family History

The lifetime risk of developing AD is greater among relatives of patients with AD.[8] Some studies have shown that at least through the middle of the ninth decade of life, relatives of patients with age of onset of AD greater than or equal to 85 years have a lower risk for AD than relatives of patients with earlier-onset AD.[9] A study done by Zintl and colleagues[10] to test the prevalence of a positive family history among dementia patients with onset before age 70 years found that of 210 patients with dementia, about 83 patients had a positive family history of dementia. A recent study involving 715 patients found that compared with patients who had no parents with AD or other types of dementia, patients who had one or both parents with AD or other types of dementia were more significantly likely to experience memory loss.[11] In this study, the patients with one or both parents with AD or other types of dementia performed poorly in verbal and visual memory tasks. Familial AD has the strongest impact on increased risk of early-onset AD, such as if one has a first-degree family member who had onset of AD before age 65 years.

Depression

Depression has been shown to be a possible risk factor for AD.[12] Studies have shown that depression symptoms are significantly associated with AD even when the onset of depression symptoms preceded the onset of identified AD symptoms by 25 years or more, and the association is much stronger among the families in which the onset of depression symptoms occurred in the year before the onset of AD symptoms.[13] Modrego and Fernandez[14] followed up 114 patients with amnestic mild cognitive impairment during a mean period of 3 years. They found that as compared with nondepressed patients with amnestic mild cognitive impairment, statistically significantly more of the depressed patients with amnestic mild cognitive impairment developed dementia of Alzheimer type, and also at an earlier age.

Education

Low educational attainment may be associated with a higher risk of AD.[15] Several prevalence surveys have reported an increased prevalence of AD in poorly educated people.[16] An increased risk of AD was found by Stern and colleagues[17] in subjects with less than 8 years of schooling. According to the cognitive reserve model, higher levels of education compensate for the neuropathology of AD, delaying its clinical manifestations. Also, as compared with less-educated people, people with higher levels of education are less likely to show clinical symptoms of dementia. Paradise and colleagues[18] reviewed the relationship between more education and decreased survival in people with AD and found that education does delay the onset of the dementia syndrome in AD but does not lead to earlier death after diagnosis.

C-Reactive Protein

Inflammation is postulated to play a role in the development of AD.[19] C-reactive protein (CRP) is a highly sensitive nonspecific marker of inflammation. Cross-sectional studies have reported elevated blood levels of CRP in patients with AD compared with control subjects.[20] Prospectively, increased levels of CRP have been associated with an increased risk of dementia 25 years later.[21] Serum CRP levels of 305 participants from a longitudinal cohort study of people aged 90 years and older were evaluated with respect to all-cause dementia. Levels of CRP were undetectable (<0.5 mg/dL), detectable (0.5–0.7 mg/dL), or elevated ($\geq$0.8 mg/dL). The results showed that in the oldest old, high CRP levels are associated with increased risk of all-cause dementia.[22] Elevated CRP levels can often be lowered by low doses of antiinflammatory drugs, such as low-dose aspirin, and so this is also a potentially modifiable risk factor.

Homocysteine

Elevated total homocysteine levels have been associated with an increased risk of atherosclerotic sequelae, including death from cardiovascular causes and clinical stroke.[23,24] If this hypothesis is valid, it points to a modifiable risk factor because plasma homocysteine levels can be lowered by supplementation with folic acid.[25] A prospective observational study involving 1092 people showed that increased plasma homocysteine level is a strong, independent risk factor for the development of dementia and AD.[26] It is not clear, however, if an elevation in plasma homocysteine concentration is a risk factor with a direct pathophysiologic role in the development of the disease or merely a risk marker reflecting an underlying process such as oxidative stress/free radical toxicity responsible for the high plasma homocysteine concentrations and the development of AD.[27]

Smoking

Studies have shown that smoking increases the risk of AD.[28] In one study, about 6870 people aged 55 years and older were followed up for a mean period of about 2.1 years and results showed that when compared with people who never smoked, people who were smokers had an increased risk of dementia and AD.[29] After assessing the same population after a longer mean follow-up period of 7.1 years, it was found that the risk of dementia with current smoking was greater in people without the apolipoprotein E-epsilon 4 (*APOE4*) allele than in *APOE4* carriers.[30] A recent meta-analysis of 19 prospective studies showed that compared with people who never smoked, people who smoked had an increased risk of dementia and decline in cognitive abilities.[31]

Diabetes

Studies have shown that diabetes may be associated with an increased risk of developing AD and a decline in cognitive function.[32] A review of longitudinal population-based studies revealed that diabetes is associated with an increased risk of AD, vascular dementia, and dementia overall.[33] Diabetes may accelerate several processes implicated in brain ageing, such as oxidative stress, accumulation of advanced glycosylation end products, microvascular dysfunction, and alterations in cerebral glucose and insulin metabolism.[34] Accelerated brain ageing in diabetes, as reflected in increased cerebral atrophy, may thus reduce the threshold for the development of AD symptoms. Also diabetes may interfere with cerebral amyloid and tau metabolism.[35]

Hyperlipidemia

Studies have shown that hypercholesterolemia may increase the risk of dementia.[36] Epidemiologic studies have established an association between higher dietary intake of saturated fats, transunsaturated fats, or cholesterol and cognitive decline and/or incident and vascular dementia.[37,38] A Cochrane review was done of double-blind randomized placebo-controlled trials of statins in people at risk of AD and dementia.[39] The results show that there is good evidence that statins given in late life to individuals at risk of vascular disease have no effect in preventing AD or dementia. It was also felt that the promising initial evidence from observational studies could have been due to selection bias.

Genetic Risk Factors

Early-onset AD is generally diagnosed if onset occurs consistently before 60 to 65 years of age and often before 55 years of age. Mutations in 3 causative genes, for example, presenilin-1, presenilin-2, and amyloid precursor protein (APP), can lead to early-onset AD.[40] Mutations in the presenilin-1 gene account for 30% to 70% of early-onset AD, mutations in the APP gene account for 10% to 15% of early-onset AD, and mutations in the presenilin-2 gene account for less than 5% of early-onset AD.[41]

APOE4 genotype is a significant risk factor for the development of late-life nonfamilial AD.[42] Corder and colleagues[43] demonstrated a dose effect of the inheritance of APOE4 on the distribution of age of onset in familial AD. Each APOE4 allele inherited increases risk and lowers the distribution of the age of onset. In a series of familial AD families, sporadic AD patients, and case controls, Corder and colleagues[44] also showed that the inheritance of an APOE2 allele decreases the risk and increases the mean age of onset.

Diet

Studies have shown that high intakes of total fat, saturated fat, and total cholesterol increase the risk of incident dementia.[37] Several epidemiologic studies have linked reduced levels of omega-3 fatty acids or fish consumption in the diet to an increased risk for age-related cognitive decline and dementia such as AD.[45] When compared with people with low caloric intake, people with a higher caloric intake may have an increased risk of developing AD.[46]

Hypertension

Studies have shown that high blood pressure may be associated with an increased risk of dementia.[47] High blood pressure may cause cerebral small-vessel pathology and hippocampal atrophy, which contributes to cognitive decline in patients with AD.[48] Alternatively, in persons with hypertension, increased numbers of neurofibrillary tangles and amyloid plaques at autopsy have also been observed, suggesting direct links between blood pressure and AD. Long-term antihypertensive treatment has been shown to decrease the incidence of AD and vascular or mixed dementia.[49]

Mental and Physical Activity

Low participation in intellectual and physical activities in midlife may be a risk factor for the later development of AD.[50] In a clinical study, more than 700 older adults underwent annual clinical evaluations for up to 5 years.[51] At baseline, they rated current and past frequency of cognitive activity with the current activity measure administered annually thereafter. During the follow-up, 90 people developed AD. Results showed that a cognitively inactive person was 2.6 times more likely to develop AD than a cognitively active person, and this association remained after controlling for past cognitive activity, lifespan, socioeconomic status, current social and physical activity, and low baseline cognitive function. Thus, cognitive inactivity in old age may be associated with increased risk of AD.

Head Trauma

Studies have shown that a history of head trauma, particularly with loss of consciousness, may be a risk factor for AD.[52] Studies have also shown that the influence of head injury on the risk of AD seems to be greater among persons lacking *APOE4* compared with those having 1 or 2 *APOE4* alleles.[53] Recurrent head trauma, such as in boxers, may increase the risk of early-onset dementia.[54] Studies have also shown that recurrent concussions may increase the risk of early-onset AD in professional football players compared with the general male population.[55]

Obesity

Being obese at midlife may be a risk factor for the later development of AD.[56]

PROTECTIVE FACTORS
Family History and Genetic Loading

Patients who have no family history of dementia may have a lower risk of developing dementia, including AD. Patients who do not carry the *APOE4* genotype may be at a lower risk of later-life onset AD than those who are carriers. Also, patients who are carriers of the *APOE2* allele seem to have a decreased risk of developing AD.[44]

Mediterranean Diet

The Mediterranean diet is a diet rich in fresh fruits, vegetables, whole grains, seafood, and olive oil. The association between adherence to the Mediterranean diet and a lower risk of AD was examined by prospectively following up 2258 individuals living in the community. They were assessed every 1.5 years. It was found that a higher adherence to the Mediterranean diet was associated with a reduction in the risk for AD.[57]

Physical Activity

Engaging in high levels of physical activity, such as exercising 3 or more times per week, has been shown to be associated with a reduced risk of AD.[58] The potential mechanism by which physical activity may have protective effects on cognition could be by sustaining cerebral blood flow by decreasing blood pressure, enhancing cerebral metabolic activity, or lowering lipid levels.[59] Recent studies have shown that compared with physically inactive individuals, physically active individuals were associated with a lower risk of AD.[60]

Education and Intellect

Higher education and occupational attainment may provide a cognitive reserve against dementia, helping to cope with advanced pathologic changes of the disease more effectively by maintaining function longer.[17,61] By this mechanism, higher education and occupational attainment may reduce the risk of AD, or delay its onset.

Brain Stimulating Activity

Longitudinal studies have shown that various types of intellectually stimulating activities may be associated with a reduced risk of dementia. Daily mentally oriented stimulating activities were associated with a decreased risk of all-cause dementia.[62] Recent follow-up studies have shown that mentally stimulating activities at work during midlife were associated with a lower risk of dementia and that highly complex mentally stimulating activity at work during midlife was associated with a lower dementia risk even among those with lower education.[63]

Cardiovascular Risk Factors

Studies have shown that hypertension treatment in old age may reduce the risk of later cognitive decline and dementia.[49] As mentioned earlier, studies have shown that diabetes is associated with an increased risk of dementia, and therefore consistent control of diabetes may prevent or delay the development of dementia in these patients. An observational study involving 301 patients with AD with and without cerebrovascular disease was done to evaluate whether the treatment of vascular risk factors, such as high blood pressure, dyslipidemia, diabetes, and atherosclerotic disease, was associated with a slower rate of cognitive decline. Results showed that patients who had their vascular risk factors treated had lesser cognitive decline than those who did not.[64] Treatment of cardiovascular risk factors may be protective and this mechanism may be an optimal control for these risk factors and direct neuroprotective effects.

PREVIOUS DEMENTIA RISK PREDICTOR STUDIES

In a study, 1409 individuals were studied in midlife and reexamined 20 years later for signs of dementia.[65] Results showed that on the follow-up after 20 years, 4% had dementia. The dementia risk score used in this study predicted significantly well those who would develop dementia. The factors involved in this score were age ($\geq$ 47 years), low education of less than 10 years, and vascular risk factors of hypertension, hypercholesterolemia, and obesity. However, there were limitations to this study. The score is applicable to the prediction of dementia risk over the next 20 years only in middle-aged people who survive for the next 20 years. People who died before the examination done at 20 years' follow-up had worse risk factor profiles than the survivors, and this survival bias could have affected the results of this study.

In another recently published study, 3375 participants with a mean age of 75 years and without evidence of dementia at baseline were identified.[66] Factors most predictive of developing incident dementia within 6 years were identified. These subjects were followed up for a period of 6 years. Factors that were found to be most predictive of dementia were included in the late-life DRI, and these were factors such as older age, worse cognitive function, body mass index less than 18.5, one or more *APOE4* alleles, slow physical performance, and magnetic resonance imaging evidence of white matter disease or enlarged ventricles. The risk of dementia was found to be less than 5% in those with low scores on this late-life DRI and more than 50% in those with high scores. However, this study had limitations because the dementia status was determined retrospectively by an adjudication committee of experts and the predictive accuracy could have been greater using other variables such as change in cognitive function.

SUMMARY

There are several risk factors for the development of dementia, including AD, as there are protective factors that may protect against its development (**Table 1**). The authors are working on developing the Saint Louis University DRI. In this risk index, one would get plus points for having 1 or more of the protective factors, such as adherence to the Mediterranean diet or having no family history of AD, and negative points for having one of the risk factors, such as higher age or less education. However, it is challenging to develop this risk index at this time, because it is not known which risk factors and protective factors are more important and which are less important.

Weighing the relative contribution/importance of individual risk and protective factors has delayed the development of a DRI. As the authors struggle to develop

Table 1		
Risk and protective factors for AD—potential mechanisms		
Factor	**Risk**	**Potential Mechanisms**
Advanced age	Increased risk	Possible decreased brain reserves
Sex	Females have increased risk	Living longer and loss of neuroprotective effects of estrogen.
Family history	Increased risk	APP, presenilin-1, presenilin-2 mutations may result in over-secretion of amyloid β (Aβ) in familial AD. APOE4 allele increases risk of sporadic (late-onset) AD
Depression	Increased risk	May decrease brain reserves/transmitters
High-fat and cholesterol diet	Increased risk	Increased neuroinflammation; possible increased substrate for APP
CRP	Increased risk	Increased neuroinflammation
Homocysteine	Increased risk	Increased oxidative stress, free radical toxicity, increased atherosclerotic sequelae
Smoking	Increased risk	Accelerated cerebral atrophy, perfusional decline, and white matter lesions
Diabetes mellitus	Increased risk	Impaired glucose uptake in neuronal cells, decreased blood supply due to small-vessel disease
Hyperlipidemia	Increased risk	Increased Aβ accumulation
Genetic	Increased risk	Mutations of presenilin-1, presenilin-2, APP
Hypertension	Increased risk	Decreased cerebral blood flow/cerebral ischemia, white matter lesions
Head trauma	Increased risk	Not fully understood. Possible blood-brain barrier disruption
Obesity	Increased risk	Hyperlipidemia and hypertension and via their mechanisms described earlier
Mediterranean diet	Decreased risk	Decreased neuroinflammation, decreased oxidative stress, decreased $A\beta_{42}$ toxicity
Increased education	Decreased risk	Education may increase neural connections
Increased mental activity	Decreased risk	Cognitive reserve model in which people cope better and can generate more neurons during their lifetime
Increased physical activity	Decreased risk	Increased cerebral blood flow, increased brain-derived neurotrophic factor

a meaningful DRI, it is becoming apparent that there are many modifiable risk and protective factors. It is important that we educate at-risk patients and family members of those with dementia about the importance of addressing modifiable factors as early as possible so as to potentially delay or decrease the risks of developing dementias such as AD. Truly, prevention is the wave of the future in the dementia arena.

REFERENCES

1. McDowell I. Alzheimer's disease: insight from epidemiology. Aging (Milano) 2001; 13(3):143–62.
2. Alzheimer's Association. Early onset dementia: a national challenge, a future crisis. Washington, DC: Alzheimer's Association; 2006. Available at: www.alz. org. Accessed June 6, 2006.
3. Gallo JJ, Lebowitz BD. The epidemiology of common late-life mental disorders in the community: themes for the new century. Psychiatr Serv 1999;50(9): 1158–66.
4. Gao S, Hendrie HC, Hall KS, et al. The relationships between age, sex, and the incidence of dementia and Alzheimer's disease: a meta-analysis. Arch Gen Psychiatry 1998;55(9):809–15.
5. Andersen K, Launer LJ, Dewey ME, et al. Gender differences in the incidence of AD and vascular dementia. The EURODEM studies. EURODEM incidence research group. Neurology 1999;53(9):1992–7.
6. Cankurtaran M, Yavuz BB, Cankurtaran ES, et al. Risk factors and type of dementia: vascular or Alzheimer? Arch Gerontol Geriatr 2008;47(1):25–34.
7. Fernandez Martinez M, Castro Flores J, Perez de Las Heras S, et al. Risk factors for dementia in the epidemiological study of Munguialde County (Basque Country-Spain). BMC Neurol 2008;8:39.
8. Huff FJ, Auerbach J, Chakravarti A, et al. Risk of dementia in relatives of patients with Alzheimer's disease. Neurology 1988;38(5):786–90.
9. Silverman JM, Smith CJ, Marin DB, et al. Familial patterns of risk in very late-onset Alzheimer's disease. Arch Gen Psychiatry 2003;60:190–7.
10. Zintl M, Schmitz G, Hajak G, et al. ApoE genotype and family history in patients with dementia and cognitively intact spousal controls. Am J Alzheimer's Dis Other Demen 2009;24:349–52.
11. Sudha Seshadri. Family history raises Alzheimers risk. American Academy of Neurology's 61st Annual Meeting. Seattle, Washington, USA. April 25 to May 2, 2009.
12. Devanand DP, Sano M, Tang MX, et al. Depressed mood and the incidence of Alzheimer's disease in the elderly living in the community. Arch Gen Psychiatry 1996;53(2):175–82.
13. Green RC, Cupples LA, Kurz A, et al. Depression as a risk factor for Alzheimer disease: the MIRAGE Study. Arch Neurol 2003;60(5):753–9.
14. Modrego PJ, Ferrandez J. Depression in patients with mild cognitive impairment increases the risk of developing dementia of Alzheimer type. Arch Neurol 2004; 61:1290–3.
15. Letenneur L, Gilleron V, Commenges D, et al. Are sex and educational level independent predictors of dementia and Alzheimer's disease? Incidence data from the PAQUID project. J Neurol Neurosurg Psychiatr 1999;66(2):177–83.
16. Katzman R. Education and the prevalence of dementia and Alzheimer's disease. Neurology 1993;43(1):13–20.

17. Stern Y, Gurland B, Tatemichi TK, et al. Influence of education and occupation on the incidence of Alzheimer's disease. JAMA 1994;271(13):1004–10.
18. Paradise M, Cooper C, Livingston G. Systematic review of the effect of education on survival in Alzheimer's disease [review]. Int Psychogeriatr 2009;21(1): 25–32.
19. Turner RS. Alzheimer's disease. Semin Neurol 2006;26(5):499–506.
20. Mancinella A, Mancinella M, Carpinteri G, et al. Is there a relationship between high C-reactive protein (CRP) levels and dementia. Arch Gerontol Geriatr 2009; 49(Suppl 1):185–94.
21. Schmidt R, Schmidt H, Curb D, et al. Early inflammation and dementia: a 25-year follow-up of the Honolulu-Asia aging study. Ann Neurol 2002;52:168–74.
22. Kravitz BA, Corrada MM, Kawas CH. Elevated C-reactive protein levels are associated with prevalent dementia in the oldest-old. Alzheimers Dement 2009;5(4): 318–23.
23. Bots ML, Launer LJ, Lindemans J, et al. Homocysteine, atherosclerosis and prevalent cardiovascular disease in the elderly: the Rotterdam Study. J Intern Med 1997;242:339–47.
24. Bostom AG, Rosenberg IH, Silbershatz H, et al. Nonfasting plasma total homocysteine levels and stroke incidence in elderly persons: the Framingham Study. Ann Intern Med 1999;131:352–5.
25. Wald DS, Bishop L, Wald NJ, et al. Randomized trial of folic acid supplementation and serum homocysteine levels. Arch Intern Med 2001;161:695–700.
26. Seshadri S, Beiser A, Selhub J, et al. Plasma homocysteine as a risk factor for dementia and Alzheimer's disease. N Engl J Med 2002;346:476–83.
27. Seshadri S. Elevated plasma homocysteine levels: risk factor or risk marker for the development of dementia and Alzheimer's disease? J Alzheimers Dis 2006; 9(4):393–8.
28. Merchant C, Tang MX, Albert S, et al. The influence of smoking on the risk of Alzheimer's disease. Neurology 1999;52(7):1408–12.
29. Ott A, Slooter AJ, Hofman A, et al. Smoking and risk of dementia and Alzheimer's disease in a population-based cohort study: the Rotterdam Study. Lancet 1998; 351(9119):1840–3.
30. Reitz C, Den Heijer T, Van Duijn C, et al. Relation between smoking and risk of dementia and Alzheimer disease: the Rotterdam Study. Neurology 2007;69(10): 998–1005.
31. Anstey KJ, von Sanden C, Salim A, et al. Smoking as a risk factor for dementia and cognitive decline: a meta-analysis of prospective studies. Am J Epidemiol 2007;166(4):367–78.
32. Arvanitakis Z, Wilson RS, Bienias JL, et al. Diabetes mellitus and risk of Alzheimer disease and decline in cognitive function. Arch Neurol 2004;61(5):661–6.
33. Biessels GJ, Staekenborg S, Brunner E, et al. Risk of dementia in diabetes mellitus: a systemic review. Lancet Neurol 2006;5(1):64–74.
34. Biessels GJ, Van der Heide LP, Kamal A, et al. Ageing and diabetes: implications for brain function. Eur J Pharmacol 2002;441(1–2):1–4.
35. Gasparini L, Xu H. Potential roles of insulin and IGF-1 in Alzheimer's disease. Trends Neurosci 2003;26(8):404–6.
36. Solomon A, Kareholt I, Ngandu T, et al. Serum cholesterol changes after midlife and late-life cognition: twenty-one-year follow-up study. Neurology 2007;68(10): 751–6.
37. Engelhart MJ, Geerlings MI, Ruitenberg A, et al. Diet and risk of dementia. Does fat matter?: the Rotterdam Study. Neurology 2002;59(12):1915–21.

38. Reitz C, Tang MX, Luchsinger J, et al. Relation of plasma lipids to Alzheimer disease and vascular dementia. Arch Neurol 2004;61(5):705–14.
39. McGuinness B, Craig D, Bullock R, et al. Statins for the prevention of dementia [review]. Cochrane Database Syst Rev 2009;(2):CD003160.
40. Hsiung GY, Sadovnick AD. Genetics and dementia: risk factors, diagnosis and management. Alzheimers Dement 2007;3:418–27.
41. Li H, Wetten S, Li L, et al. Candidate single-nucleotide polymorphisms from a genomewide association study of Alzheimer disease. Arch Neurol 2008;65(1): 45–53.
42. Gene tests. Available at: www.genetests.org. Accessed April 30, 2009.
43. Corder EH, Saunders AM, Strittmatter WJ, et al. Gene dose of apolipoprotein E type 4 allele and the risk of Alzheimer's disease in late onset families. Science 1993;261:921–3.
44. Corder EH, Saunders AM, Risch NJ, et al. Protective effect of apolipoprotein E type 2 allele for late onset Alzheimer disease. Nat Genet 1994;7:180–4.
45. Cole GM, Ma QL, Frautschy SA. Omega-3 fatty acids and dementia. Prostaglandins Leukot Essent Fatty Acids 2009;81(2–3):213–21.
46. Luchsinger JA, Tang MX, Shea S, et al. Caloric intake and the risk of Alzheimer disease. Arch Neurol 2002;59(8):1258–63.
47. Whitmer RA, Sidney S, Selby J, et al. Midlife cardiovascular risk factors and risk of dementia in late life. Neurology 2005;64(2):277–81.
48. Den Heijer T, Launer LJ, Prins ND, et al. Association between blood pressure, white matter lesions, and atrophy of the medial temporal lobe. Neurology 2005; 64(2):263–7.
49. Forette F, Seux ML, Staessen JA, et al. The prevention of dementia with antihypertensive treatment: new evidence from the Systolic Hypertension in Europe (Syst-Eur) study. Arch Intern Med 2002;162(18):2046–52 [Erratum in: Arch Intern Med 2003;163(2):241].
50. Friedland RP, Fritsch T, Smyth KA, et al. Patients with Alzheimer's disease have reduced activities in midlife compared with healthy control-group members. Proc Natl Acad Sci U S A 2001;98(6):3440–5.
51. Wilson RS, Scherr PA, Schneider JA, et al. Relation of cognitive activity to risk of developing Alzheimer's disease. Neurology 2007;69(20):1911–20.
52. Plassman BL, Havlik RJ, Steffens DC, et al. Documented head injury in early adulthood and risk of Alzheimer's disease and other dementias. Neurology 2000;55(8):1158–66.
53. Guo Z, Cupples LA, Kurz A, et al. Head injury and the risk of AD in the MIRAGE study. Neurology 2000;54(6):1316–23.
54. Mendez MF. The neuropsychiatric aspects of boxing. Int J Psychiatry Med 1995; 25(3):249–62.
55. Guskiewicz KM, Marshall SW, Bailes J, et al. Association between recurrent concussion and late-life cognitive impairment in retired professional football players. Neurosurgery 2005;57(4):719–26 [discussion: 719–26].
56. Whitmer RA, Gunderson EP, Quesenberry CP Jr, et al. Body mass index in midlife and risk of Alzheimer disease and vascular dementia. Curr Alzheimer Res 2007; 4(2):103–9.
57. Scarmeas N, Stern Y, Tang MX, et al. Mediterranean diet and risk for Alzheimer's disease. Ann Neurol 2006;59(6):912–21.
58. Laurin D, Verreault R, Lindsay J, et al. Physical activity and risk of cognitive impairment and dementia in elderly persons. Arch Neurol 2001;58(3):498–504.

59. Rogers RL, Meyer JS, Mortel KF. After reaching retirement age physical activity sustains cerebral perfusion and cognition. J Am Geriatr Soc 1990;38:123–8.
60. Scarmeas N, Luchsinger JA, Schupf N, et al. Physical activity, diet and risk of Alzheimer disease. JAMA 2009;302(6):627–37.
61. Stern Y, Tang MX, Denaro J, et al. Increased risk of mortality in Alzheimer's disease patients with more advanced educational and occupational attainment. Ann Neurol 1995;37:590–5.
62. Wang HX, Karp A, Winblad B, et al. Late-life engagement in social and leisure activities is associated with a decreased risk of dementia: a longitudinal study from the Kungsholmen project. Am J Epidemiol 2002;155(12):1081–7.
63. Karp A, Andel R, Parker MG, et al. Mentally stimulating activities at work during midlife and dementia risk after age 75: follow-up study from the Kungsholmen Project. Am J Geriatr Psychiatry 2009;17(3):227–36.
64. Deschaintre Y, Richard F, Leys D, et al. Treatment of vascular risk factors is associated with slower decline in Alzheimer disease. Neurology 2009;73(9):674–80.
65. Kivipelto M, Ngandu T, Laatikainen T, et al. Risk score for the prediction of dementia risk in 20 years among middle aged people: a longitudinal, population-based study. Lancet Neurol 2006;5(9):721.
66. Barnes DE, Covinsky KE, Whitmer RA, et al. Predicting risk of dementia in older adults: The late-life dementia risk index. Neurology 2009;73(3):168–9.

Potential Future Neuroprotective Therapies for Neurodegenerative Disorders and Stroke

Rawan Tarawneh, MD[a,b], James E. Galvin, MD, MPH[a,b,c,d],*

KEYWORDS

- Parkinson disease • Alzheimer disease • Ischemic stroke
- Amyotrophic lateral sclerosis • Huntington disease

The cellular mechanisms underlying neuronal loss and neurodegeneration have been an area of interest in the last decade. Although neurodegenerative diseases such as Alzheimer disease (AD), Parkinson disease (PD), Huntington disease (HD), and amyotrophic lateral sclerosis (ALS) each have specific pathologies, they all share common mechanisms such as protein aggregation, oxidative injury, neuroinflammation, apoptosis, and mitochondrial injury that contribute to neuronal loss. Current research in these areas has focused on developing neuroprotective therapies that target each of these mechanisms. Studies from animal and cell models have greatly expanded our knowledge in this field and form the basis of clinical trials of neuroprotective therapies. Results have been variable; it is likely that no single therapy will be satisfactory, and that multiple agents working through different mechanisms or novel agents that target more than one disease mechanism may offer the best hope for a future neuroprotective therapy. This review addresses several mechanisms of disease pathogenesis in

This study was supported by grants P01 AG03991 and P50 AG05681 from the National Institute on Aging.

[a] Alzheimer Disease Research Center, Washington University School of Medicine, 4488 Forest Park Avenue, Suite 130, St Louis, MO 63108, USA
[b] Department of Neurology, Washington University School of Medicine, St Louis, MO 63108, USA
[c] Department of Psychiatry, Washington University School of Medicine, St Louis, MO 63108, USA
[d] Department of Neurobiology, Washington University School of Medicine, St Louis, MO 63108, USA
* Corresponding author. Alzheimer Disease Research Center, Washington University School of Medicine, 4488 Forest Park Avenue, Suite 130, St Louis, MO 63108.
E-mail address: galvinj@neuro.wustl.edu (J.E. Galvin).

neurodegenerative disease and stroke (**Table 1**), along with some examples of therapies targeting each of these mechanisms. Although the authors have attempted to provide a comprehensive review of the available literature, inclusion of all studies and hypotheses in this area is beyond the scope of this review.

TARGETING SPECIFIC MECHANISMS OF DISEASE PATHOGENESIS
Oxidative Stress

PD

The substantia nigra (SN) of PD contains high levels of reactive oxygen species (ROS) such as superoxide and perioxynitrites in conjunction with a high iron content associated with neuromelanin,[1] and reduced levels of antioxidant mechanisms such as glutathione and uric acid.[2,3] The mitochondrial toxin 1-methyl-4-phenyl-1,2,3,6-tetrahydropyridine (MPTP) blocks the mitochondrial electron transport chain by inhibiting complex I,[4] and several abnormalities in complex I and IV have been implicated in PD.[5] Oxidative stress and mitochondrial dysfunction may be interrelated in a self-propagating circle.[6] Inhibition of complex I leads to excess production of the ROS that target the electron transport chain, resulting in the formation of further increased amounts of toxic radicals.[6] Furthermore, the metabolism of dopamine itself creates a favorable environment for oxidative damage through intermediates such as dopamine quinone and 3,4-diydroxyphenylacetaldehyde.[7]

Several compounds with antioxidant properties have been studied as potential neuroprotective agents in PD. One open label study of vitamin E 3200 IU/d and vitamin C 3000 mg/d suggested that the time to levodopa (L-Dopa) was delayed by 2.5 years,[8] whereas the Deprenyl and Tocopherol Anti-Oxidative Therapy of Parkinsonism (DATA-TOP) trial of vitamin E and deprenyl (selegiline)[9] showed no benefit for vitamin E, but a modest protective effect and slowing of disease progression with deprenyl.[10] In one clinical trial (TEMPO),[11] patients initiated on the monoamine oxidase B (MAO$_B$) inhibitor rasagiline at baseline were improved at 1 year compared with patients initiated on placebo and switched to rasagiline at 6 months. Results from a larger randomized trial of rasagiline monotherapy (1 or 2 mg/d) in mild PD (the ADAGIO [Attenuation of Disease Progression with Rasagiline Once-Daily] trial) were recently reported.[12] Early treatment with rasagiline at a dose of 1 mg, but not 2 mg, per day provided benefits that were consistent with a possible disease-modifying effect.[12]

Oral coenzyme Q10 (CoQ10) 1200 mg/d was shown to slow motor deterioration, and improve activities of daily living in a 16-month randomized trial of patients with mild PD.[13] Experimental animal models of PD using a toxic hydroxylated analog of dopamine 6-hydroxydopamine (6-OHDA) suggest that the detrimental effects of this

Table 1
Potential targets for novel therapies
Oxidative stress
Excitotoxicity
Inflammation
Mitochondrial dysfunction
Apoptosis
Protein misfolding/aggregation
Neurotrophic factors
Gene therapy

compound can be blocked by the use of iron-chelating compounds, MAO_B inhibitors, and antioxidants such as vitamin E.[14] In a small open pilot study, the use of glutathione 600 mg intravenously (IV) twice daily in patients with PD resulted in a significant decrease in their disability scores.[15]

AD

Increased peroxidation of membrane lipids, DNA, RNA, and protein have all been described in AD. Oxidative stress is involved in amyloid-β (Aβ) toxicity; in vitro oxidation of soluble Aβ promotes its transformation into the aggregated form, creating a vicious cycle of aggregation and oxidative damage. There is in vivo evidence that amyloid aggregation can be inhibited by antioxidants, and in vitro studies suggest that the free radical scavengers, vitamin E and propyl gallate, protect neuronal cells against Aβ toxicity.[16]

Results of clinical trials regarding the benefit of vitamin E and C on the risk of AD have been conflicting. Supplementary intake of vitamin E or C was associated with better cognitive performance in one study.[17] A large 6-year follow-up study suggests that dietary intake of vitamin E is associated with a lower risk for developing AD, particularly in smokers, and irrespective of the apolipoprotein E genotype.[18] On the other hand, other studies failed to show such a benefit, although vitamin E may be associated with delayed time to death, institutionalization, loss of ability to perform basic activities, and severe dementia.

In addition to vitamins, numerous free radical scavengers have been used in experimental paradigms of neuronal cell death in vitro and in vivo, such as the pineal hormone melatonin, the potent lipid peroxidation inhibitors known as the 21-aminosteroids or lazaroids, mifepristone (RU486), and the female sex hormone estrogen. Early melatonin administration reduces antioxidant stress and inhibits apoptosis in animal models of AD.[19] Lazaroids such as the U-74,006F or tirilazad mesylate can attenuate the increased lipid peroxidation observed in AD.[20] Another series of antioxidants, the 2-methylaminochromans such as the compound U-78,517F, may be more potent and effective inhibitors of lipid peroxidation than the 21-aminosteroids.[21]

Stroke

Radical scavengers (such as vitamin E, sulfhydryl compounds, and nitrone spin traps), agents that promote detoxification of ROS (superoxide dismutase, catalase, or peroxidase conjugates), and agents that prevent radical generation (eg, the xanthine oxidase inhibitor allopurinol, nitric oxide synthase inhibitors, or nonsteroidal antiinflammatory agents and cyclooxygenase inhibitors) have been studied in stroke. The use of NXY-059 has been associated with clinical benefits in animal models of stroke, and was associated with a significant improvement in the modified Rankin functional scale in the Stroke-Acute Ischemic NXY Treatment-I (SAINT-I) trial.[22] However, these results were not reproduced in the expanded SAINT-II trial.[23,24] Ebselen and the radical scavenger edaravone (MCI-186, Radicut) were associated with clinical improvement in a small trial.[25]

HD

Antioxidants that have shown potential benefit in animal models of HD include thiol, the mitochondrial enzyme cofactor lipoic acid, and the combination of vitamin E and Q10.[26] Treatment with Q10 was associated with reduced levels of 8-hydroxyguanosine (a marker of oxidative damage) and improved survival in R6/2 mice. There was a trend toward slowing decline in total functional capacity, although these did not reach clinical significance in a large clinical trial of Q10.[27] A randomized trial of vitamin E in HD showed no benefit, although post hoc analyses suggest a possible benefit in early disease.[28]

Excitotoxicity and N-Methyl-D-Aspartate Glutamate Receptors

Excessive N-methyl-D-aspartate (NMDA) receptor activation has been implicated in the pathophysiology of several neurodegenerative diseases and in stroke.

PD

Following the loss of dopamine, enhanced NMDA receptor-mediated transmission in the striatum may be part of the cascade of events leading to the generation of parkinsonian symptoms. The dopaminergic deficit results in enhanced activity of the subthalamic nucleus and increased glutaminergic output to the basal ganglia.[29] Studies on dopamine denervated rats and MPTP-treated parkinsonian monkeys have provided insight into the relative abundance of different NMDA subunits in the striatum. Dopamine depletion in the 6-OHDA rat models and MPTP primate models results in relative decreases in the abundance of NMDA receptor subtype 1 (NR1) and subtype 2B (NR2B) subunits in the synaptosomal membranes, which is restored by chronic L-Dopa therapy.[30,31] Because stimulation of NR2B-containing NMDA receptors contributes to the generation of parkinsonian symptoms,[32] NR2B-selective NMDA receptor antagonists may be therapeutically beneficial for parkinsonian patients. Prior administration of NMDA receptor antagonist dizocilpine MK-801 suppresses the dopa-induced increase in glutamate in 6-hydroxydopamine-lesioned rats and may therefore offer neuroprotection.[33]

Several NMDA antagonists have been studied in PD. Amantadine and dextromethorphan have antidyskinetic effects, and amantadine is associated with increased lifespan.[34,35] On the other hand, memantine did not show any benefit in one trial.[36] Selective NMDA receptor antagonists, such as ifenprodil and CP-101,606, have been developed in an attempt to avoid the side effects of nonselective blockers. Ifenprodil has antiparkinsonian actions in rat and nonhuman primates.[37–39] CP-101,606, reduced parkinsonian symptoms in haloperidol-treated rats and MPTP-lesioned nonhuman primates.[40] Pretreatment of 6-OHDA-lesioned rats with BZAD-0, 4-trifluoromethoxy-N-(2-trifluoromethyl-benzyl)-benzamidine (BZAD-01), a novel selective inhibitor of the NMDA NR1A/2B receptor, significantly reduced the amount of dopamine cell loss and significantly improved all behavioral measures.[41] When given in combination with L-Dopa-carbidopa, the NMDA antagonist remacemide has been shown to reduce parkinsonism in rodent and monkey models of PD.[42] However, it failed to demonstrate a clear benefit in clinical trials.[43] The usefulness of riluzole, a presynaptic inhibitor of glutamate release, as a neuroprotective agent in PD was addressed in a large multicenter randomized clinical trial, which was halted after preliminary results showed no evidence of a neuroprotective effect.[44]

The simultaneous blockade of AMPA (α-amino-3-hydroxy-5-methyl-4-isoxazolepropionic acid) and NMDA receptors offers substantially greater reduction in the response alterations induced by L-Dopa than inhibition of either of these receptors alone in rat and primate models of PD. Simultaneous blockade of the AMPA receptors with GYKI-47,261 and NMDA receptor with amantadine or MK-801 resulted in significant reductions in L-Dopa–induced dykinesias in a primate model, whereas the wearing-off dyskinesias were completely ameliorated in rat models of PD.[45]

AD

Several studies have linked τ and amyloid aggregation to glutamate-mediated toxicity and suggest the involvement of NMDA subunits in the pathogenesis of AD.[46] In situ hybridization studies revealed lower NR1 mRNA levels in the layer III of the entorhinal cortex and dentate gyrus in AD brains.[47] AD is associated with reduced levels of 2 mRNA isoform subsets of the NR1 receptor and changes in the expression of NR2A and NR2B in the superior temporal cortex, cingulate cortex, and hippocampus.[48] Moreover, the levels of NR1 and NR2B expression decrease with disease progression. The presence of presenilin-1 in a macromolecular complex with NR1 and NR2A further supports a role for excitotoxicity in AD.[49]

Therapeutic intervention with high-affinity NMDA receptor antagonists, such as phencyclidine (PCP) and MK-801, is not practical because of adverse side effects. Memantine is an uncompetitive NMDA receptor antagonist and can decrease pathologic activation of NMDA receptors without affecting physiologic NMDA receptor activity.[50] Memantine is associated with functional improvement in patients with AD and has been approved by the US Food and Drug Administration for the treatment of AD.[50,51]

Stroke

Excitotoxicity has been a widely investigated area in stroke. Ischemic neuronal injury in vitro depends on synaptic release of excitatory amino acids (EAAs) and resultant elevation of intracellular free calcium. Even transient exposure to excess excitatory amino acids is toxic to cultured neurons, and alterations in neuronal energy balance increases the vulnerability of neurons to excitotoxic damage even in the presence of physiologic concentrations of EAAs.[52] Evidence that this process progresses for several hours after the ischemic insult highlights a potential role for neuroprotective strategies administered during the critical window before irreversible loss, although the exact duration of this window in humans remains unknown. The action of glutamate on NMDA receptors seems to play an important role in glutamate-mediated toxicity. Compounds that decrease glutamate levels or interfere with its binding to this receptor have been the focus of many studies.[53]

NMDA antagonists that have been investigated in stroke include aptiganel hydrochloride (CNS 1102, Cerestat), dextrorphan, and dextromethorphan. Their use was associated with side effects and no clear clinical benefit in clinical trials.[52] Phase II trials of oral and IV forms of remacemide hydrochloride in stroke are currently under way. Magnesium ion, which electrophysiologically behaves as a noncompetitive NMDA antagonist, has demonstrated efficacy as a neuroprotective agent in focal and global models of cerebral ischemia. Two preliminary trials of IV magnesium show no evidence of adverse effects,[54,55] and phase III trials are currently under way. A phase II trial of Selfotel (CGS 19755) in patients with acute stroke reported evidence of a dose-dependent toxicity.[56] Selective NMDA antagonists such as ifenprodil and eliprodil (SL82.0715) have demonstrated preclinical neuroprotective efficacy, and eliprodil is currently being investigated in early phase III trials in patients with stroke. Other compounds under investigation are 3-(2-carboxypiperazin-4-yl)-propyl-1-phosphonic acid (CPP), its derivative d-CPPene, and CGS 19,755.[57] Neuroprotection is evident for the presynaptic glutamate release inhibitors 619C89 and lubeluzole when administered within 6 hours of induced ischemia. Both drugs are currently in phase II trials in stroke.

Partial glycine agonists, such as HA 966, L687414, and 1-aminocyclopropanecarboxylic acid (ACPC), or full antagonists, such as 7-chlorokynurenic acid and its derivatives or ACEA 1021, are effective in stroke models. Glutamate antagonists at other receptor subtypes, such as the AMPA receptors, are under evaluation.[52]

HD

Injections of EAAs into the striatum of rodents and primates results in neuronal death and a neurologic phenotype similar to that of HD. Intrastriatal injections of NMDA glutamate agonists, such as quinolinic acid, have been used to create animal models of HD. Animal models and human studies show evidence of decreased glutamate receptors, in particular the mGluR2 subtypes, downregulation of the GLT-1 glial glutamate transporter, and increased sensitization of NMDA receptors.[58]

The efficacy of memantine in slowing down the rate of progression was studied in a 2-year, open, and multicenter trial with promising results.[59] Cannabinoid-derived drugs also offer promise in protecting neurons from glutamate mediate toxicity. Activation of neuronal CB(1) or CB(2) cannabinoid receptors attenuates excitotoxic glutamatergic neurotransmission and triggers prosurvival signaling pathways. The administration of CB(2) receptor-selective agonists reduced neuroinflammation, brain edema, striatal neuronal loss, and motor symptoms in wild-type mouse models subjected to excitotoxicity.[60]

Inflammation

PD

There is evidence that systemic inflammation may promote microglial activation in PD, and genes implicated in PD may also influence inflammatory mediators.[61] Overexpression of wild-type α-synuclein in neurons is associated with the activation of microglia, and the release of tumor necrosis factor (TNF), interleukin 1β (IL-1β), IL-6, cyclooxygenase (COX)-2, and inducible nitric oxide synthase (iNOS).[62] Animal models of PD using MPTP also show evidence of recruitment of CD4 T cells to the SN.[63]

Minocycline, a tetracycline derivative, has been shown to reduce microglial activation and inhibit the release of potentially toxic cytokines in the striatal region of MPTP mice. Pretreatment with minocycline improved survival of dopaminergic SN neurons in animal models of PD.[64] The use of nonaspirin nonsteroidal antiinflammatory agents has been associated with a 45% reduction in the risk of developing PD in one prospective study with 14 years of follow-up.[65] Cytokines (particularly TNF-α) activate COX-1 and COX-2, which catalyze the conversion of arachidonic acid to prostaglandins and thromboxanes. Mixed COX-1/COX-2 inhibitors and selective COX-2 inhibitors were shown to partially protect against MPTP-induced striatal depletion in rodents.[66] Further preclinical studies are needed in this area.

AD

Several inflammatory mediators may have a role in the pathogenesis of AD. In a prospective cohort study of subjects with AD, acute systemic inflammatory events were associated with an increase in the serum levels of proinflammatory cytokines[67] and a 2-fold increase in the rate of cognitive decline over a 6-month period. High baseline levels of TNF-α were also found to be associated with a 4-fold increase in the rate of cognitive decline.

Clinical studies suggest that nonsteroidal antiinflammatory drugs cause a delay in the onset or slow down progression of AD, through the inhibition of COX and lipooxygenases, and resultant decrease in prostaglandin synthesis and ROS formation.[68] In vitro studies of neuronal cell lines have shown that glutathione depletion induces the activation of neuronal 12-lipoxygenase (12-LOX), which leads to the production of peroxides, the influx of Ca^{2+}, and ultimately to cell death.[69] Exposure to glutamate is associated with induction of the enzyme COX-2, suggesting a possible role for COX inhibitors in neuroprotection.[70] Compounds with antiinflammatory activity such as glucocorticoids, antimalaria drugs, and colchicines are potential areas of interest. Treatment with a moderate dose of prednisone has been shown to suppress serum levels of acute phase proteins in patients with AD.[71] The neurohormone melatonin exerts inhibitory effects on β-amyloid aggregation, oxidation, and inflammation in vitro, and results in behavioral improvement in animal models.[72]

The peroxisome proliferator-activated receptor (PPAR) plays an important role in regulating the expression of enzymes involved in lipid metabolism. Specific PPAR isoforms have been shown to suppress the expression of the proinflammatory cytokines IL-1, TNF, and IL-6 and decrease the activity of the transcription factors of NF-κB, AP-1, and STAT proteins. Activation of PPARα results in decreased differentiation of monocytes into activated macrophages, decreased β-amyloid-stimulated expression of IL-6 and TNF-α, and decreased expression of COX-2.[73]

Stroke

Several inflammatory mediators such as leukocytes, adhesion molecules, acute phase reactants, cytokines, and proteases are increased in the plasma of patients with cerebral ischemia. The early central inflammatory events include the production of ROS (eg, nitric oxide and superoxide), expression of proteolytic enzymes (matrix metalloproteinase [MMP]-9 and MMP-2), vasoactive substances (prostaglandins and cyclooxygenases), and vascular adhesion molecules (intercellular adhesion molecule 1 [ICAM-1], P-selectin, and L-selectin). Neutrophils and macrophages are considered early contributors to the production of ROS and cytokines, whereas activation of microglia and proliferation of astrocytes in the ischemic area further promote the inflammatory response in later stages.[74]

Inflammatory mediators (such as IL-1β, IL-6, TNF-α, IL-10, transforming growth factor beta [TGF-β] and chemokines including membrane cofactor protein 1 (MCP-1), macrophage inflammatory protein 1 [MIP-1], keratinocyte-derived chemokine/chemokine [CXC motif] ligand 1/[KC/CXCL1] and fractalkine [CX3CL1]) are also found in increased levels in brain tissue in animal models of stroke. The expression of IL-1β mRNA is increased in the ischemic rat brain within hours after the induction of stroke,[75] increased levels of IL-6 are seen in the plasma and cerebrospinal fluid 3 to 6 hours after experimental stroke in mice,[76] and levels of proinflammatory cytokines such as IL-6, interferon-γ (IFN-γ), and MCP-1 become increased in the plasma within 6 hours in rodents.[77]

The anti-ICAM-1 antibody, enlimomab, can reduce the size of stroke when given within 1 hour of reperfusion after transient, but not permanent ischemia, in a rat stroke model. However, its use was associated with significant worsening in the modified Rankin scale and higher mortality at 90 days compared with placebo in a large clinical trial.[78] Blocking neutrophil activation by a recombinant protein inhibitor of the CD11b/CD18 receptor, UK 279,276 (Rovelizumab), within 6 hours of stroke also failed to show any benefits in one clinical trial, which was stopped prematurely. Despite promising results for IL-1 receptor antagonist in several animal studies, this drug has not been investigated in humans.[79] FK506 also demonstrates benefits, particularly after transient ischemia, in animal studies and remains a potential target for studies in humans.[80] Systemic administration of minocycline is protective in experimental models of focal[81] or global[82] cerebral ischemia. Inhibition of IL-1β converting enzyme[83] or deletion of IL-1β and IL-1α results in markedly reduced ischemic damage and neuronal death in animal studies.[84] Deficiency of inflammatory chemokines such as MCP-1[85] or fractalkine[86] is associated with less vulnerability to ischemic injury.

HD

Neuroinflammation is a prominent feature associated with HD and may constitute a novel target for neuroprotection. Increased expression of several key inflammatory mediators, including chemokine (c-c motif) ligand 2 (CCL2) and IL-10, has been reported in the striatum of patients with HD. There is also evidence of upregulation of IL-6, IL-8, and MMP9, in the cortex and notably the cerebellum.[87] Minocycline can reduce calpain-mediated inflammation and caspase-dependent neurodegeneration, and was found to be neuroprotective in HD rat models. However, it cannot effectively prevent calpain-dependent neuronal death in cell culture models.[88]

Mitochondrial Dysfunction

PD

Perhaps, the most convincing evidence for the role of mitochondrial damage in PD comes from studies of rare familial forms of PD, in which genetic mutations linked to PD result in mitochondrial impairments and increased susceptibility to oxidative stress. For example, *Parkin* knockouts demonstrate impaired mitochondrial activity and altered oxidative stress proteins in mouse and *Drosophila* models.[89,90] Disruption of DJ-1, a mitochondrial protein with antioxidant chaperone activity, and mutations in PTEN-induced kinase (PINK1),[91] are associated with impaired mitochondrial and proteosomal functions.[92]

Creatine is a precursor of the energy intermediate phosphocreatine, and transfers phosphoryl groups for adenosine triphosphate (ATP) synthesis in mitochondria. Dietary supplementation of carnitine resulted in decreased loss of dopaminergic cells in an MPTP mouse model of PD,[93,94] possibly through the modulation of the Ras/ NF-κB signaling pathway. CoQ10 provides significant protection against MPTP-induced dopamine depletion.[95–97] A significant reduction in CoQ10 levels in mitochondria has been reported in the platelets of patients with PD, and directly correlates with a decrease in complex I activity. In one study, the oral administration of CoQ10 in patients with PD resulted in significant dose-dependent increases in plasma CoQ10 levels, and a statistically significant dose-dependent reduction in Unified Parkinson Disease Rating Scale scores compared with placebo. MitoQ contains coenzyme Q10 (CoQ10) covalently linked to the lipophilic cation triphenylphosphonium. MitoQ helps preserve mitochondrial function after glutathione depletion,[98] and is currently in a phase II clinical trial for PD (http://www.parkinsons.org.nz/news/protectstudy. asp). Preliminary data also suggest that SS-31 and SS-20 (antiapoptotic mitochondrial proteins referred to as Szeto-Schiller [SS] proteins) produce complete protection against MPTP neurotoxicity.[99] Others such as carnitine, β-hydroxybutyrate, and nicotinamide have been shown to protect against MPTP-induced neurodegeneration in mice.

AD

Alterations in mitochondrial size, structure, and function have been extensively reported in AD. These include deficiency in enzymes involved in oxidative metabolism (such as α-ketoglutarate dehydrogenase complex, and pyruvate dehydrogenase complex), altered calcium homeostasis, and sporadic mtDNA rearrangements. Amyloid precursor protein (APP) accumulates in mitochondria and levels of mitochondrial APP seem to directly correlate with mitochondrial dysfunction and severity of the disease. AD is also associated with abnormal distribution of mitochondria as they accumulate in the soma and are reduced in the neuronal processes of AD pyramidal neurons. Furthermore, synaptic dysfunction is one of the early and most robust correlates of AD-associated cognitive deficits, suggesting a role for Aβ-induced mitochondrial dysfunction in the pathogenesis of early AD.[100]

Antioxidants that specifically target mitochondria are currently being studied in AD.[101] A phase II clinical trial of the orally active antioxidant MitoQ is under way in AD. CoQ10 treatment has been shown to decrease brain oxidative stress, reduce β-amyloid plaque load, and improve cognitive performance in a transgenic mouse model of AD.[102] Creatine administration protects against glutamate and β-amyloid toxicity in rat hippocampal neurons.[103] Idebenone prevents β-amyloid-induced toxicity and, in combination with α-tocopherol, can improve β-amyloid-induced learning and memory deficits in rats.[103,104] The administration of idebenone 90 mg three times/d orally in patients with AD was associated with statistically significant improvement of memory, attention, and behavior in a multicenter trial.[105] Another randomized multicenter study trial of idebenone reported a statistically significant and dose-dependent improvement in the Alzheimer's Disease Assessment Scale (ADAS) score after 6 months.[106]

Stroke

The release of multiple apoptogenic proteins from mitochondria has been identified in ischemic and postischemic neurons. Results from animal models strongly implicate caspase-dependent and caspase-independent apoptosis and the mitochondrial permeability transition as important contributors to tissue damage, particularly when induced by short periods of temporary focal ischemia.[107] Prophylactic administration of oral creatine reduces the size of ischemic brain infarctions in mice. The antioxidant SS peptide SS-31 plays an important role in modulating ROS-induced mitochondrial permeability transition and cell death, and has been found to be protective in several in vitro and in vivo models of ischemia and reperfusion injury. Synthetic triterpenoids are analogs of oleanolic acid, which exert antioxidative effects through stimulation of the antioxidant response element Nrf2-Keap1 signaling pathway, and have been shown to be protective in a rat model of cerebral ischemia.[98]

HD

HD is associated with significant defects in mitochondrial respiratory enzymes, including mitochondrial succinate dehydrogenase (SDH, complex II) and aconitase. Protein aggregates interfere with mitochondrial function, mitochondrial trafficking in axons, and result in mitochondrial fragmentation and inhibition of mitochondrial fusion. SDH inhibitors, including 3-nitropropionic acid and malonate cause medium spiny neuronal loss and clinical and pathologic features reminiscent of HD in rodents and nonhuman primates.[98]

Results from studies on HD transgenic mice suggest that high-dose CoQ10 significantly extends survival, improves motor performance and grip strength, and reduces brain atrophy in R6/2 HD mice in a dose-dependent manner. The combination of CoQ10 and minocycline in an R6/2 mouse model of HD resulted in significantly improved behavioral measures, reduced neuropathologic deficits, extended survival, and attenuated striatal neuronal atrophy, compared with either agent alone.[108] Similarly, the combination of CoQ10 and remacemide (NMDA antagonist) resulted in significantly improved motor performance and increased survival in the R6/2 and the N171-82Q transgenic mouse models of HD.[109] These 2 compounds were studied separately and in combination in 340 patients with HD. Administration of CoQ10 resulted in a 14% decrease in disease progression, whereas remacemide demonstrated no efficacy.[27]

Creatine significantly improves survival, improves motor performance, increases brain ATP levels, and delays atrophy of striatal neurons and the formation of Htt-positive aggregates in the R6/2 and N171-82Q transgenic mouse models of HD.[110] Idebenone was not associated with significant improvement in a small trial in HD.[111] A phase III trial of 2400 mg of CoQ10 daily has recently started in HD, and a phase II trial of CoQ10 in presymptomatic gene-positive patients with HD (PREQUEL) will begin soon.[112]

PPARγ co-activator 1α (PGC-1α) is a transcriptional regulator of several enzymes such as the nuclear respiratory factors 1 and 2, Tfam, and estrogen-related receptor α involved in mitochondrial biogenesis. Potential usefulness of this factor in neuroprotection has been suggested by reports of impaired expression in HD transgenic mice and patients with HD. PGC-1α induced the expression of antioxidant enzymes and its overexpression is associated with protection of neural cells from the oxidation by mitochondrial toxins.[113] Sirtuins (silent information regulators) are members of the NAD$^+$-dependent histone deacetylase family of proteins in yeast and play an important role in regulating mitochondrial function. Inhibition of sirtuins has been shown to suppress disease pathogenesis in *Drosophila* models of HD.[114] SIRT1 activation by resveratrol has been associated with increased survival of motor neurons from transgenic ALS mice.[115] In AD, SIRT1 activation by resveratrol significantly protects against microglia-dependent A-β toxicity by inhibiting NF-κB signaling and is associated with cognitive improvement in AD mouse models.[115]

Apoptosis

In general, antiapoptotic strategies under evaluation for neuroprotection include strategies to prevent caspase-dependent apoptosis (eg, caspase inhibitors) or strategies to prevent caspase-independent apoptosis (eg, poly(adenosine diphosphate ribose) polymerase [PARP] inhibitors).

PD

Dopaminergic cells in PD exhibit increased expression of the proapoptotic protein Bax and effector protease caspase-3 compared with controls.[116] Significantly higher levels of caspase-8 activation have been demonstrated in the dopaminergic neurons of SN pars compacta of patients with PD compared with controls,[117] and caspase-8 activation occurs early after exposure to cellular toxins such as 1,2,3,6-tetrahydropyridine in in vivo experimental animal models of PD. Patients with untreated PD have high peripheral levels of caspase-3 activity in lymphocytes and upregulation of antiapoptotic Bcl-2, which correlate with disease duration and severity. Treatment with L-Dopa and dopamine agonists is associated with lower levels of antiapoptotic Bcl-2 in the blood, and higher densities of the peripheral benzodiazepine receptor.[118]

CEP-1347 is an inhibitor of mixed lineage kinases, which in turn regulate the c-jun N-terminal kinase pathway (JUNK) pathway. CEP-1347 has been shown to enhance neuronal survival in cell models of PD. However, it failed to show efficacy in the early treatment of PD in one clinical study.[119] Minocycline has been shown to block MPTP-induced dopamine depletion in the striatum, decreases inducible NO synthase and caspase-1 expression, and inhibits NO-induced phosphorylation of p38 mitogen-activated protein kinase. TCH 346 (*N*-methyl-*N*-propargyl-10-aminomethyl-dibenzo[*b*,-*f*]oxepin [also referred to as CGP3466]) is a potent antiapoptotic drug that has been shown to prevent the loss of dopaminergic neurons in vitro, and protect against behavioral abnormalities and neurodegeneration in animal models of PD.[120] This novel drug is believed to block the transcriptional upregulation of protective molecules such as Bcl-2 and superoxide dismutase.[120] However, it failed to demonstrate efficacy as a neuroprotective agent in 1 randomized placebo controlled trial.[121]

Studies of caspase inhibitors in animal models of PD have led to mixed results. The peptidyl inhibitor carbobenzoxy-Val-Ala-Asp-fluoromethylketone (zVADfmk) can protect neurons from apoptosis induced by mitochondrial toxins. However, its therapeutic efficacy is limited by its poor penetrability into the brain.[122] The more potent broad-spectrum caspase inhibitor, Q-VD-OPH, may be more promising. Specific caspase inhibitors, such as acetyl-tyrosinyl-valyl-alanyl-aspartyl-chloromethylketone

(Ac-YVAD-cmk), have also demonstrated efficacy in several experimental paradigms of PD.[123] On the other hand, other studies have found no benefit with caspase inhibitors. The treatment of 1-methyl-4-phenylpyridinium-intoxicated primary dopaminergic cultures with broad-spectrum and specific caspase-8 inhibitors triggered a switch from apoptosis to necrosis, with no overall neuroprotective benefits in one study.[117] Further studies are needed in this area.

Propargylamines have proven to be potent antiapoptotic agents in in vitro and in vivo studies, as these peptides can prevent mitochondrial permeabilization, cytochrome c release, caspase activation, and nuclear translocation of glyceraldehyde-3-phosphate dehydrogenase.[124] In fact, inhibition of apoptosis through caspase inhibition may underlie the action of the propargylamine-derived MAO_B inhibitors such as rasagiline and deprenyl (selegiline).[125] Moreover, rasagiline seems to induce antiapoptotic prosurvival proteins, Bcl-2, and glial cell line–derived neurotrophic factor.[126] In addition to its symptomatic benefits as a dopaminergic agent, selegiline has been shown to delay the need for symptomatic therapy in patients with untreated PD in the DATATOP study.[9] Lazabemide is a reversible inhibitor of MAO_B that is not a propargylamine. Results from a randomized double blinded study suggested a delay in the need for L-Dopa treatment and a possible neuroprotective benefit. However, studies of this compound have been discontinued by the sponsor.

AD

The activation of PARP plays a critical role in caspase-independent apoptosis. Therefore, PARP inhibitors represent one possible therapeutic strategy in AD. PARP-1 has been implicated in DNA repair and maintenance of genomic integrity. The generation of ROS causes overactivation of PARP, resulting in the depletion of NAD(+) and ATP, and consequently in necrotic cell death and organ dysfunction.[127]

There is evidence to suggest that apoptosis is associated with senile plaques containing Aβ peptide in AD brains, and this effect may be mediated through ROS. The effect of Pycnogenol (PYC), a potent antioxidant and ROS scavenger, on Aβ(25–35)-induced apoptosis was investigated in an animal model of AD. PYC suppressed the generation of ROS, caspase-3 activation, DNA fragmentation, PARP cleavage, and eventually protected against Aβ-induced apoptosis. A significant increase in ROS formation preceded apoptotic events after the cells were exposed to Aβ (25–35).[128]

HD

Several lines of evidence point to a role for apoptosis in animal models and in postmortem tissue of HD. Caspase-3 has been shown to cleave mutant huntingtin and the activation of caspase-1 has been reported in the HD brain. The expression of expanded polyglutamine residues has been associated with apoptotic mechanisms via caspase activation and cleavage of the death substrates lamin B and inhibitor of caspase-activated DNase (ICAD).[129] Bax expression in peripheral B and T lymphocytes and monocytes is increased in HD, and lymphoblasts derived from patients with HD show increased stress-induced apoptotic cell death associated with caspase-3 activation.[130]

Recent findings suggest a possible role for the hypoxia-inducible factor 1 (HIF-1) in HD. HIF-1 regulates the expression of several genes, including mediators of apoptosis, making it a potential target for future therapies.[131] Extracellular ATP stimulates apoptosis through stimulation of P2X7 receptors, and subsequent alterations in calcium permeability, both of which have been described in HD. The in vivo administration of the P2X7-antagonist Brilliant Blue-G to HD mice prevented neuronal apoptosis and attenuated motor coordination deficits.[132]

Stroke

Caspase-dependent and caspase-independent mechanisms of cell death are implicated in focal cerebral ischemia. Increased expression of Fas and of mediators of the extrinsic caspase-dependent pathway have been shown following focal ischemia. Increased expression of caspase-1, -3, -8, and -9, and of cleaved caspase-8, has been observed in the penumbra. The role for apoptosis in ischemia is further supported by reports that the inhibition of caspase-3 reduces infarct size after transient focal ischemia.[133]

Intranuclear MMP activity facilitates oxidative injury in neurons during early ischemia through the cleavage of PARP-1 and XRCC1, and resultant disturbance of DNA repair mechanisms. Inhibition of MMP with the broad-spectrum inhibitor BB1101 significantly attenuated ischemia-induced PARP-1 cleavage, and resultant cell death in a rat model of focal cerebral ischemia.[134] The p53-dependent receptor pathway also seems to be involved in stroke-induced apoptosis. Injection of netrin-1, a ligand of the receptor uncoordinated gene 5H2 (UNC5H2), was associated with significantly reduced infarct volume at 3 days after focal ischemia in an animal model of stroke, through its inhibition of p53-mediated apoptosis.[135] Estrogen has also been shown to prevent Fas-mediated apoptosis in experimental models of stroke.[136]

Misfolding of Protein and Protein Aggregation

PD

Several animal studies and studies of familial PD have shown that the overexpression of the wild-type and the mutant forms of α-synuclein can lead to loss of dopaminergic terminals, the aggregation of α-synuclein and subsequently to motor impairment. On the other hand, α-synuclein knockouts do not display any characteristic phenotype other than minor deficits in dopamine transmission.[137] Lentiviral-mediated expression of wild-type rat α-synuclein in rats resulted in the formation of aggregates but no cell loss.[138] Based on these results, it is plausible that either misfolded α-synuclein , or increased amounts of normal α-synuclein, contribute to neurotoxicity in PD. Other studies have demonstrated the presence of large amounts of α-synuclein aggregates in the presynaptic region terminals. These occur in parallel with significant synaptic pathology and may, at least partially, account for the discrepancy between the number of neocortical Lewy bodies and the degree of neuronal loss or cognitive impairment.[139]

Much of our current understanding of possible ways to target the accumulation of α-synuclein in α-synucleinopathies has been based on studies of amyloid aggregation in patients with AD. Animal and in vitro cell models suggest that the conversion of some amyloidogenic proteins from random structure to a β-sheet-rich aggregated form can be inhibited by the addition of peptides derived from the respective amyloidogenic protein.[140] Previous studies on the use of peptide inhibitors in AD by the insertion of an N-methylated amino acid to provide a β-sheet-breaking peptide provided the basis for the development of methylated α-synuclein as a potential target in PD and Lewy body dementia.[141] The formation of an N-methylated derivative of synuclein, by the replacement of the Gly73 with sarcosine, resulted in reduced fibril formation and markedly reduced toxicity.[142,143]

α-Synuclein peptide fragments that bind to full-length α-synuclein have also been studied as potential targets for inhibiting α-synuclein aggregation. Peptides derived from the N-terminal of the nonamyloidogenic component region of α-synuclein can bind to the full-length α-synuclein and block the assembly of α-synuclein into early oligomers and mature amyloidlike fibrils. Furthermore, the addition of a polyarginine-peptide delivery system has allowed the development of a cell permeable inhibitor of aggregation, the peptide RGGAVVTGRRRRR-amide, which inhibits iron-induced DNA damage in cells transfected with α-synuclein (A53T).[143,144] A novel and potentially disease-modifying approach to α-synuclein-related disorders includes the inhibition of α-synuclein filament assembly with molecular compounds such as β-synuclein-derived small peptides.[145] The fibrillization of the murine α-synuclein can be inhibited by human α-synuclein, with a possible role for at least 1 of the 6 mismatched residues between the 2 proteins, most of which were located in the C terminal region.[146] Along this line, β-synuclein is a nonamyloidogenic homolog of α-synuclein and has been characterized as an inhibitor of α-synuclein aggregation either by direct interactions or indirect inhibitory effects on the accumulation of toxic α-synuclein oligomers.[145] Several catecholamines, including dopamine, have been shown to exhibit inhibitory effects on α-synuclein fibrillization depending on their state of oxidation and to lead to the accumulation of α-synuclein protofibrils.[147]

AD

Potential inhibitors of Aβ aggregation include rifampicin, 5,8-dihydroxy-3R-methyl-2R-(dipropylamino)-1,2,3,4-tetrahydronaphthalene, type IV collagen, melatonin, daunomycin, glycosaminoglycans, fullerene, apomorphine derivatives, 3-indole propionic acid, nordihydroguaiaretic acid, tannic acid, 3-amino-1-propanesulfonic acid (Alzhemed or Tramiposate), salvianolic acid B, and Δ^9-tetrahydrocannabinol among others.

Several reports have shown that peptides or peptidomimetics can inhibit Aβ aggregation. Peptides that incorporate N-methylated amino acids in critical positions exert such an effect. N-methylated derivatives of the aggregation-prone fragment of Aβ, Aβ-(25-35), have been shown to prevent Aβ-(25-35) aggregation and inhibit toxicity in PC12 cells. N-methylated peptides of other regions of the peptides, such as Aβ-(36–40) may also effectively inhibit aggregation. PPI-1019 D-(His-[(mLeu)-Val-Phe-Phe-Leu]-NH$_2$) is another effective N-methylated peptide inhibitor of Aβ aggregation and toxicity, which uses the methylation of an amine, rather than amide, in the unacetylated N-terminus.[148] The efficacy of these agents in inhibiting aggregation is sensitive to minor changes in testing conditions. However, the translation of these findings into development of disease-modifying therapies is less than straightforward. Drug development of compounds such as Alzhemed and iAβ5p has been discontinued.

Similarly, there has been a search for inhibitors of τ aggregation. Methylene blue was the first such substance identified, followed by several anthraquinones such as daunorubicin and Adriamycin. Anthraquinone analogs can reduce the formation of τ inclusions in neuroblastoma cells that overexpress a 4R human τ fragment. Other inhibitors include phenothiazines, porphyrins, and polyphenols.[149] Several N-phenylamine, phenylthiazolylhydrazide, and rhodanine compounds have been added to the list of the τ aggregation inhibitors of interest.

HD

Expression of several molecular chaperones such as Hsp70, Hsp40, Hsp27, Hsp84, and Hsp105 has been shown to increase the solubility of polyQ proteins in *Drosophila* and mouse disease models. In vitro studies show that Hsp70 and Hsp40 promote the formation of soluble unstructured aggregates. The Hsp90 inhibitor geldanamycin, and its less toxic derivative 17-demethoxygeldanamycin (17-AAG), increase the expression of molecular chaperones, thereby preventing the aggregation of the polyQ protein in cell culture and animal models.

Intracellular antibodies (intrabodies) that target polyQ protein and prevent its aggregation have been identified. These include the intrabody C4, which recognizes the

N-terminal region of huntingtin protein (htt), and intrabodies MW7 and VL 12.3, which recognize regions adjacent to the polyQ stretch of htt. These antibodies can inhibit inclusion body formation in cell cultures and prevent neurodegeneration in *Drosophila* and yeast models of HD. Other peptides, such as polyglutamine binding peptide 1-6 (QBP1-6) and QBP1 (SNWKWWPGIFD), can interfere with the conformational changes associated with aggregation. Peptides consisting of 2 normal-length polyQ stretches connected by a spacer have been developed that can break β-pleated sheets and inhibit their aggregation, although they may be less effective than QB1.[150]

Orally administered molecules that can mimic the therapeutic effects of biomolecules offer another potential area for development of polyQ aggregation inhibitors. Benzothiazole derivatives, including PGL-135, offered promise in vitro and in cell culture; however, these results were not reproduced in mouse models. The green tea polyphenol (-)-epigallocatechin-3-gallate (EGCG) can potently inhibit htt aggregation in vitro and in a *Drosophila* model of HD. Similarly, compounds that can stabilize the native conformation may be useful in preventing aggregation. Examples of these include dimethyl sulfoxide, glycerol, trimethylamine *N*-oxide, and trehalose. Using a yeast model-based high-throughput screening assay, thousands of similar compounds have been identified and need to be evaluated in larger studies.[150]

Growth Factors and Gene Therapies

Several trophic factors have been shown to protect dopaminergic neurons when given before exposure to toxins, in in vivo and in vitro models of PD. Only a few, such as glial cell line–derived neurotrophic factor (GDNF) and its relative, neurturin (NRTN, also known as NTN), have been shown to promote restoration of neurons in the aftermath of a toxic exposure, therefore making them potential therapeutic candidates for PD.[151,152] However, their use has been limited by lack of effective means of delivery into the selected cell population; GDNF delivered by intracerebroventricular injection in patients had limited penetration into the putamen, and intraputaminal infusions were ineffective, probably because of limited distribution within the putamen.[152] Gene therapies use a viral vector to deliver a protein of interest to specific brain regions and may be useful as a means of delivery of tropic factors.[153] Preliminary results from a phase II randomized clinical trial with gene therapy for NRTN, using adeno-associated virus to deliver the trophic factor to the striatum, have recently been presented (http://www.ceregene.com/).

GPI-1485 and NIL-A belong to the group of neuroimmunophilins, compounds that are derived from the immunosuppressant FK 506 (tacrolimus), but have no immunosuppressant function. Neuroimmunophilins exhibit neurotrophic effects in animal models of PD, and can easily cross the blood-brain barrier. Their exact mechanism of action is unknown, but may involve indirect stimulation of neurotrophic factor production. The results of clinical trials with these compounds have been insignificant. GPI-1046 is another neuroimmunophilin that is under development.[154,155] GM-1 ganglioside, a constituent of cell membranes, has been shown to facilitate the neurotrophic action of GDNF and brain-derived neurotrophic factor (BDNF) and inhibit apoptosis in in vivo and in vitro models of PD. Phase I studies of this compound seem to be promising.[125]

Stem cells are pluripotential cells that offer the potential of generating unlimited numbers of optimized dopamine cells for transplantation. Stem cells can be grown and expanded in tissue culture and then induced to differentiate into dopamine neuronal phenotypes. Transplantation of these cells into the striatum has been associated with behavioral improvement in 6-OHDA rodents and MPTP monkeys.[156] Results of fetal cell transplant have been inconclusive, with conflicting results regarding the survival of the grafts,[157–159] and questions remain regarding the optimization of selective dopaminergic cell transplantation.[160]

AD

Hippocampal neural stem cell transplantation has been shown to improve the spatial learning and memory deficits in aged transgenic mice without altering Aβ or τ pathologic conditions. This beneficial effect seems to be mediated through BDNF and resultant enhancement of hippocampal synaptic density.[161]

Estrogen modulates the expression of neurotrophic factors, such as nerve growth factor, enhances a nonamyloidogenic processing of APP, and prevents apoptosis. Observational evidence implies that use of hormone therapy at a younger age close to the time of menopause may reduce the risk of AD later in life, although initiation of estrogen therapy during late postmenopause has been associated with increased risk for dementia. Trials to address this issue are under way (Early versus Late Intervention Trial with Estrogen; Kronos Early Estrogen Prevention Study).[162] Neurosteroid alloprognanolones (APα) are potent proliferative agents that can promote neurogenesis in vitro and in vivo of rodent and human neural stem cells, and are being studied in AD.

HD

Trophic factors such as Tr-κB, the receptor for BDNF, have been investigated as potential neuroprotective agents in HD. The ciliary neurotrophic factor and BDNF have a benefit in vivo in mouse models of HD. However, their use in clinical trials depends on the development of delivery methods to the brain such as the use of encapsulated cells or viral-mediated expression. Cysteamine, a candidate drug for HD, has been shown to increase BDNF levels in the brain and to induce neuroprotection in HD mouse models.[150]

SUMMARY

This review describes the depth and breadth of possible targets for the therapeutic intervention of diverse diseases such as PD, AD, HD, and stroke. Although each of these disorders has different causes, clinical and cognitive symptoms, disease course, duration, progression, and pathologic conditions, the underlying pathways subserving these diverse disorders share common targets. Most of these approaches will not make it to phase III clinical trials. However, in a short period of roughly 40 years from the introduction of L-Dopa for the symptomatic treatment of PD, 20 years of thrombolytic therapies for stroke, and 15 years of symptomatic treatment of AD with cholinesterase inhibitors, rapid advances in molecular biology and genetics have opened new avenues of research including the 100 or so targets discussed in this review and the hundreds more that the authors were unable to address.

REFERENCES

1. Fasano M, Bergamasco B, Lopiano L. Modifications of the iron-neuromelanin system in Parkinson's disease. J Neurochem 2006;96:909.
2. Ihara Y, Chuda M, Kuroda S, et al. Hydroxyl radical and superoxide dismutase in blood of patients with Parkinson's disease: relationship to clinical data. J Neurol Sci 1999;170:90.
3. Sian J, Dexter DT, Lees AJ, et al. Alterations in glutathione levels in Parkinson's disease and other neurodegenerative disorders affecting basal ganglia. Ann Neurol 1994;36:348.

4. Nicklas WJ, Youngster SK, Kindt MV, et al. MPTP, MPP+ and mitochondrial function. Life Sci 1987;40:721.
5. Muftuoglu M, Elibol B, Dalmizrak O, et al. Mitochondrial complex I and IV activities in leukocytes from patients with parkin mutations. Mov Disord 2004;19:544.
6. Dauer W, Przedborski S. Parkinson's disease: mechanisms and models. Neuron 2003;39:889.
7. Jackson-Lewis V, Smeyne RJ. MPTP and SNpc DA neuronal vulnerability: role of dopamine, superoxide and nitric oxide in neurotoxicity. Minireview. Neurotox Res 2005;7:193.
8. Fahn S. A pilot trial of high-dose alpha-tocopherol and ascorbate in early Parkinson's disease. Ann Neurol 1992;32(Suppl):S128.
9. Shoulson I. DATATOP: a decade of neuroprotective inquiry. Parkinson Study Group. Deprenyl and tocopherol antioxidative therapy of Parkinsonism. Ann Neurol 1998;44:S160.
10. Olanow CW, Hauser RA, Gauger L, et al. The effect of deprenyl and levodopa on the progression of Parkinson's disease. Ann Neurol 1995;38:771.
11. Parkinson Study Group. A controlled trial of rasagiline in early Parkinson disease: the TEMPO Study. Arch Neurol 1937;59:2002.
12. Olanow CW, Rascol O, Hauser R, et al. A double-blind, delayed-start trial of rasagiline in Parkinson's disease. N Engl J Med 2009;361:1268.
13. Shults CW, Oakes D, Kieburtz K, et al. Effects of coenzyme Q10 in early Parkinson disease: evidence of slowing of the functional decline. Arch Neurol 2002;59:1541.
14. Schober A. Classic toxin-induced animal models of Parkinson's disease: 6-OHDA and MPTP. Cell Tissue Res 2004;318:215.
15. Sechi G, Deledda MG, Bua G, et al. Reduced intravenous glutathione in the treatment of early Parkinson's disease. Prog Neuropsychopharmacol Biol Psychiatry 1996;20:1159.
16. Behl C. Alzheimer's disease and oxidative stress: implications for novel therapeutic approaches. Prog Neurobiol 1999;57:301.
17. Masaki KH, Losonczy KG, Izmirlian G, et al. Association of vitamin E and C supplement use with cognitive function and dementia in elderly men. Neurology 2000;54:1265.
18. Engelhart MJ, Geerlings MI, Ruitenberg A, et al. Dietary intake of antioxidants and risk of Alzheimer disease. JAMA 2002;287:3223.
19. Cheng Y, Feng Z, Zhang QZ, et al. Beneficial effects of melatonin in experimental models of Alzheimer disease. Acta Pharmacol Sin 2006;27:129.
20. Youdim MB, Bar Am O, Yogev-Falach M, et al. Rasagiline: neurodegeneration, neuroprotection, and mitochondrial permeability transition. J Neurosci Res 2004;79:172.
21. Hall ED. Novel inhibitors of iron-dependent lipid peroxidation for neurodegenerative disorders. Ann Neurol 1992;32(Suppl):S137.
22. Lees KR, Zivin JA, Ashwood T, et al. NXY-059 for acute ischemic stroke. N Engl J Med 2006;354:588.
23. Feuerstein GZ, Zaleska MM, Krams M, et al. Missing steps in the STAIR case: a translational medicine perspective on the development of NXY-059 for treatment of acute ischemic stroke. J Cereb Blood Flow Metab 2008;28:217.
24. Shuaib A, Lees KR, Lyden P, et al. NXY-059 for the treatment of acute ischemic stroke. N Engl J Med 2007;357:562.
25. Green AR, Ashwood T. Free radical trapping as a therapeutic approach to neuroprotection in stroke: experimental and clinical studies with NXY-059 and free radical scavengers. Curr Drug Targets CNS Neurol Disord 2005;4:109.

26. Kamat CD, Gadal S, Mhatre M, et al. Antioxidants in central nervous system diseases: preclinical promise and translational challenges. J Alzheimers Dis 2008;15:473.

27. Huntington Study Group. A randomized, placebo-controlled trial of coenzyme Q10 and remacemide in Huntington's disease. Neurology 2001;57:397.

28. Peyser CE, Folstein M, Chase GA, et al. Trial of d-alpha-tocopherol in Huntington's disease. Am J Psychiatry 1995;152:1771.

29. Blandini F, Porter RH, Greenamyre JT. Glutamate and Parkinson's disease. Mol Neurobiol 1996;12:73.

30. Dunah AW, Wang Y, Yasuda RP, et al. Alterations in subunit expression, composition, and phosphorylation of striatal N-methyl-D-aspartate glutamate receptors in a rat 6-hydroxydopamine model of Parkinson's disease. Mol Pharmacol 2000;57:342.

31. Hallett PJ, Dunah AW, Ravenscroft P, et al. Alterations of striatal NMDA receptor subunits associated with the development of dyskinesia in the MPTP-lesioned primate model of Parkinson's disease. Neuropharmacology 2005;48:503.

32. Hallett PJ, Standaert DG. Rationale for and use of NMDA receptor antagonists in Parkinson's disease. Pharmacol Ther 2004;102:155.

33. Jonkers N, Sarre S, Ebinger G, et al. MK801 suppresses the L-DOPA-induced increase of glutamate in striatum of hemi-Parkinson rats. Brain Res 2002;926:149.

34. Uitti RJ, Rajput AH, Ahlskog JE, et al. Amantadine treatment is an independent predictor of improved survival in Parkinson's disease. Neurology 1996;46:1551.

35. Verhagen L, Blanchet PJ, van den Munckhof P, et al. A trial of dextromethorphan in parkinsonian patients with motor response complications. Mov Disord 1998; 13:414–7.

36. Merello M, Nouzeilles MI, Cammarota A, et al. Effect of memantine (NMDA antagonist) on Parkinson's disease: a double-blind crossover randomized study. Clin Neuropharmacol 1999;22:273.

37. Nash JE, Brotchie JM. Characterisation of striatal NMDA receptors involved in the generation of parkinsonian symptoms: intrastriatal microinjection studies in the 6-OHDA-lesioned rat. Mov Disord 2002;17:455.

38. Nash JE, Fox SH, Henry B, et al. Antiparkinsonian actions of ifenprodil in the MPTP-lesioned marmoset model of Parkinson's disease. Exp Neurol 2000;165: 136.

39. Nash JE, Hill MP, Brotchie JM. Antiparkinsonian actions of blockade of NR2B-containing NMDA receptors in the reserpine-treated rat. Exp Neurol 1999;155: 42.

40. Steece-Collier K, Chambers LK, Jaw-Tsai SS, et al. Antiparkinsonian actions of CP-101,606, an antagonist of NR2B subunit-containing N-methyl-d-aspartate receptors. Exp Neurol 2000;163:239.

41. Leaver KR, Allbutt HN, Creber NJ, et al. Neuroprotective effects of a selective N-methyl-D-aspartate NR2B receptor antagonist in the 6-hydroxydopamine rat model of Parkinson's disease. Clin Exp Pharmacol Physiol 2008;35:1388.

42. Greenamyre JT, Eller RV, Zhang Z, et al. Antiparkinsonian effects of remacemide hydrochloride, a glutamate antagonist, in rodent and primate models of Parkinson's disease. Ann Neurol 1994;35:655.

43. Shoulson I, Penney J, McDermott M, et al. A randomized, controlled trial of remacemide for motor fluctuations in Parkinson's disease. Neurology 2001;56: 455.

44. Rascol O, Olanow CW, Brooks D, et al. A 2-year multicenter placebo-controlled, double blind parallel group study of the effect of riluzole in Parkinson's disease [abstract]. Mov Disord 2002;17(Suppl 5):39.

45. Bibbiani F, Oh JD, Kielaite A, et al. Combined blockade of AMPA and NMDA glutamate receptors reduces levodopa-induced motor complications in animal models of PD. Exp Neurol 2005;196:422.

46. Koutsilieri E, Riederer P. Excitotoxicity and new antiglutamatergic strategies in Parkinson's disease and Alzheimer's disease. Parkinsonism Relat Disord 2007;13(Suppl 3):S329.

47. Mishizen-Eberz AJ, Rissman RA, Carter TL, et al. Biochemical and molecular studies of NMDA receptor subunits NR1/2A/2B in hippocampal subregions throughout progression of Alzheimer's disease pathology. Neurobiol Dis 2004;15:80.

48. Hynd MR, Scott HL, Dodd PR. Differential expression of N-methyl-D-aspartate receptor NR2 isoforms in Alzheimer's disease. J Neurochem 2004;90:913.

49. Saura CA, Choi SY, Beglopoulos V, et al. Loss of presenilin function causes impairments of memory and synaptic plasticity followed by age-dependent neurodegeneration. Neuron 2004;42:23.

50. Farlow MR, Graham SM, Alva G. Memantine for the treatment of Alzheimer's disease: tolerability and safety data from clinical trials. Drug Saf 2008;31:577.

51. Bakchine S, Loft H. Memantine treatment in patients with mild to moderate Alzheimer's disease: results of a randomised, double-blind, placebo-controlled 6-month study. J Alzheimers Dis 2008;13:97.

52. Muir KW, Lees KR. Clinical experience with excitatory amino acid antagonist drugs. Stroke 1995;26:503.

53. Nakanishi N, Tu S, Shin Y, et al. Neuroprotection by the NR3A subunit of the NMDA receptor. J Neurosci 2009;29:5260.

54. Muir KW, Lees KR. Intravenous magnesium sulphate in acute stroke: a randomised, double-blind, placebo-controlled pilot study [abstract]. Cerebrovasc Dis 1994;4:255.

55. Wester PO, Asplund K, Eriksson S, et al. Infusion of magnesium in patients with acute brain infarction [abstract]. Acta Neurol Scand 1984;70:143.

56. Clark WM, Coull BM. Randomised trial of CGS19755, a glutamate antagonist, in acute ischemic stroke treatment. Neurology 1994;44(Suppl 2):A270.

57. Taylor CP. Mechanism of action of new anti-epileptic drugs. In: Chadwick D, editor. New trends in epilepsy management: the role of gabapentin. London: Royal Socty of Medicine Services Limited; 1994. p. 13–40.

58. Leegwater-Kim J, Cha JH. The paradigm of Huntington's disease: therapeutic opportunities in neurodegeneration. NeuroRx 2004;1:128.

59. Beister A, Kraus P, Kuhn W, et al. The N-methyl-D-aspartate antagonist memantine retards progression of Huntington's disease. J Neural Transm Suppl 2004; 68:117–22.

60. Palazuelos J, Aguado T, Pazos MR, et al. Microglial CB2 cannabinoid receptors are neuroprotective in Huntington's disease excitotoxicity. Brain 2009;132(pt 11):3152–64.

61. Lee JK, Tran T, Tansey MG. Neuroinflammation in Parkinson's Disease. J Neuroimmune Pharmacol 2009. [Epub ahead of print].

62. Su X, Maguire-Zeiss KA, Giuliano R, et al. Synuclein activates microglia in a model of Parkinson's disease. Neurobiol Aging 2008;29:1690.

63. Brochard V, Combadiere B, Prigent A, et al. Infiltration of CD4+ lymphocytes into the brain contributes to neurodegeneration in a mouse model of Parkinson disease. J Clin Invest 2009;119:182.

64. Du Y, Ma Z, Lin S, et al. Minocycline prevents nigrostriatal dopaminergic neurodegeneration in the MPTP model of Parkinson's disease. Proc Natl Acad Sci U S A 2001;98:14669.

65. Chen H, Zhang SM, Hernan MA, et al. Nonsteroidal anti-inflammatory drugs and the risk of Parkinson disease. Arch Neurol 2003;60:1059.
66. Teismann P, Ferger B. Inhibition of the cyclooxygenase isoenzymes COX-1 and COX-2 provide neuroprotection in the MPTP-mouse model of Parkinson's disease. Synapse 2001;39:167.
67. Holmes C, Cunningham C, Zotova E, et al. Systemic inflammation and disease progression in Alzheimer disease. Neurology 2009;73:768.
68. Klegeris A, McGeer PL. Non-steroidal anti-inflammatory drugs (NSAIDs) and other anti-inflammatory agents in the treatment of neurodegenerative disease. Curr Alzheimer Res 2005;2:355.
69. Li Y, Maher P, Schubert D. A role for 12-lipoxygenase in nerve cell death caused by glutathione depletion. Neuron 1997;19:453.
70. Tocco G, Freire-Moar J, Schreiber SS, et al. Maturational regulation and regional induction of cyclooxygenase-2 in rat brain: implications for Alzheimer's disease. Exp Neurol 1997;144:339.
71. Aisen PS. Inflammation and Alzheimer disease. Mol Chem Neuropathol 1996;28:83.
72. Olcese JM, Cao C, Mori T, et al. Protection against cognitive deficits and markers of neurodegeneration by long-term oral administration of melatonin in a transgenic model of Alzheimer disease. J Pineal Res 2009;47:82.
73. Combs CK, Bates P, Karlo JC, et al. Regulation of beta-amyloid stimulated proinflammatory responses by peroxisome proliferator-activated receptor alpha. Neurochem Int 2001;39:449.
74. Denes A, Thornton P, Rothwell NJ, et al. Inflammation and brain injury: acute cerebral ischaemia, peripheral and central inflammation. Brain Behav Immun 2009, in press.
75. Liu T, McDonnell PC, Young PR, et al. Interleukin-1 beta mRNA expression in ischemic rat cortex. Stroke 1993;24:1746.
76. Clark WM, Rinker LG, Lessov NS, et al. Time course of IL-6 expression in experimental CNS ischemia. Neurol Res 1999;21:287.
77. Offner H, Subramanian S, Parker SM, et al. Experimental stroke induces massive, rapid activation of the peripheral immune system. J Cereb Blood Flow Metab 2006;26:654.
78. Enlimomab Acute Stroke Trial Investigators. Use of anti-ICAM-1 therapy in ischemic stroke: results of the Enlimomab acute stroke trial. Neurology 2001;57:1428.
79. Banwell V, Sena ES, Macleod MR. Systematic review and stratified meta-analysis of the efficacy of interleukin-1 receptor antagonist in animal models of stroke. J Stroke Cerebrovasc Dis 2009;18:269.
80. Macleod MR, O'Collins T, Horky LL, et al. Systematic review and metaanalysis of the efficacy of FK506 in experimental stroke. J Cereb Blood Flow Metab 2005;25:713.
81. Yrjanheikki J, Tikka T, Keinanen R, et al. A tetracycline derivative, minocycline, reduces inflammation and protects against focal cerebral ischemia with a wide therapeutic window. Proc Natl Acad Sci U S A 1999;96:13496.
82. Yrjanheikki J, Keinanen R, Pellikka M, et al. Tetracyclines inhibit microglial activation and are neuroprotective in global brain ischemia. Proc Natl Acad Sci U S A 1998;95:15769.
83. Hara H, Friedlander RM, Gagliardini V, et al. Inhibition of interleukin 1beta converting enzyme family proteases reduces ischemic and excitotoxic neuronal damage. Proc Natl Acad Sci U S A 2007;94:1997.

84. Boutin H, LeFeuvre RA, Horai R, et al. Role of IL-1alpha and IL-1beta in ischemic brain damage. J Neurosci 2001;21:5528.

85. Hughes PM, Allegrini PR, Rudin M, et al. Monocyte chemoattractant protein-1 deficiency is protective in a murine stroke model. J Cereb Blood Flow Metab 2002;22:308.

86. Soriano SG, Amaravadi LS, Wang YF, et al. Mice deficient in fractalkine are less susceptible to cerebral ischemia-reperfusion injury. J Neuroimmunol 2002;125:59.

87. Silvestroni A, Faull RL, Strand AD, et al. Distinct neuroinflammatory profile in post-mortem human Huntington's disease. Neuroreport 2009;20:1098.

88. Bantubungi K, Jacquard C, Greco A, et al. Minocycline in phenotypic models of Huntington's disease. Neurobiol Dis 2005;18:206.

89. Greene JC, Whitworth AJ, Kuo I, et al. Mitochondrial pathology and apoptotic muscle degeneration in Drosophila parkin mutants. Proc Natl Acad Sci U S A 2003;100:4078.

90. Palacino JJ, Sagi D, Goldberg MS, et al. Mitochondrial dysfunction and oxidative damage in parkin-deficient mice. J Biol Chem 2004;279:18614.

91. Valente EM, Abou-Sleiman PM, Caputo V, et al. Hereditary early-onset Parkinson's disease caused by mutations in PINK1. Science 2004;304:1158.

92. Deng H, Jankovic J, Guo Y, et al. Small interfering RNA targeting the PINK1 induces apoptosis in dopaminergic cells SH-SY5Y. Biochem Biophys Res Commun 2005;337:1133.

93. Bender A, Koch W, Elstner M, et al. Creatine supplementation in Parkinson disease: a placebo-controlled randomized pilot trial. Neurology 2006;67:1262.

94. NINDS NET-PD Investigators. A randomized, double-blind, futility clinical trial of creatine and minocycline in early Parkinson disease. Neurology 2006;66:664.

95. Faust K, Gehrke S, Yang Y, et al. Neuroprotective effects of compounds with antioxidant and anti-inflammatory properties in a Drosophila model of Parkinson's disease. BMC Neurosci 2009;10:109.

96. Shults CW, Haas RH, Beal MF. A possible role of coenzyme Q10 in the etiology and treatment of Parkinson's disease. Biofactors 1999;9:267.

97. Young AJ, Johnson S, Steffens DC, et al. Coenzyme Q10: a review of its promise as a neuroprotectant. CNS Spectr 2007;12:62.

98. Chaturvedi RK, Beal MF. Mitochondrial approaches for neuroprotection. Ann N Y Acad Sci 2008;1147:395.

99. Yang L, Zhao K, Calingasan NY, et al. Mitochondria targeted peptides protect against 1-methyl-4-phenyl-1,2,3,6-tetrahydropyridine neurotoxicity. Antioxid Redox Signal 2009;11(9):2095–104.

100. Su B, Wang X, Zheng L, et al. Abnormal mitochondrial dynamics and neurodegenerative diseases. Biochim Biophys Acta 2010;1802(1):135–42.

101. Bolognesi ML, Matera R, Minarini A, et al. Alzheimer's disease: new approaches to drug discovery. Curr Opin Chem Biol 2009;13:303.

102. Kipiani K, Dumont M, Yu F, et al. Coenzyme Q10 decreases amyloid pathology and improves behavior in a transgenic mouse model of Alzheimer's disease. Neurobiol Dis 2009, in press.

103. Brewer GJ, Wallimann TW. Protective effect of the energy precursor creatine against toxicity of glutamate and beta-amyloid in rat hippocampal neurons. J Neurochem 2000;74:1968.

104. Yamada K, Tanaka T, Han D, et al. Protective effects of idebenone and alpha-tocopherol on beta-amyloid-(1-42)-induced learning and memory deficits in rats: implication of oxidative stress in beta-amyloid-induced neurotoxicity in vivo. Eur J Neurosci 1999;11:83.

105. Weyer G, Babej-Dolle RM, Hadler D, et al. A controlled study of 2 doses of idebenone in the treatment of Alzheimer's disease. Neuropsychobiology 1997; 36:73.

106. Gutzmann H, Hadler D. Sustained efficacy and safety of idebenone in the treatment of Alzheimer's disease: update on a 2-year double-blind multicentre study. J Neural Transm Suppl 1998;54:301.

107. Sims NR, Muyderman H. Mitochondria, oxidative metabolism and cell death in stroke. Biochim Biophys Acta 2010;1802(1):80–91.

108. Stack EC, Smith KM, Ryu H, et al. Combination therapy using minocycline and coenzyme Q10 in R6/2 transgenic Huntington's disease mice. Biochim Biophys Acta 2006;1762:373.

109. Ferrante RJ, Andreassen OA, Dedeoglu A, et al. Therapeutic effects of coenzyme Q10 and remacemide in transgenic mouse models of Huntington's disease. J Neurosci 2002;22:1592.

110. Andreassen OA, Dedeoglu A, Ferrante RJ, et al. Creatine increases survival and delays motor symptoms in a transgenic animal model of Huntington's disease. Neurobiol Dis 2001;8:479.

111. Ranen NG, Peyser CE, Coyle JT, et al. A controlled trial of idebenone in Huntington's disease. Mov Disord 1996;11:549.

112. Shults CW, Haas R. Clinical trials of coenzyme Q10 in neurological disorders. Biofactors 2005;25:117.

113. McGill JK, Beal MF. PGC-1alpha, a new therapeutic target in Huntington's disease? Cell 2006;127:465.

114. Pallos J, Bodai L, Lukacsovich T, et al. Inhibition of specific HDACs and sirtuins suppresses pathogenesis in a *Drosophila* model of Huntington's disease. Hum Mol Genet 2008;17:3767.

115. Kim D, Nguyen MD, Dobbin MM, et al. SIRT1 deacetylase protects against neurodegeneration in models for Alzheimer's disease and amyotrophic lateral sclerosis. EMBO J 2007;26:3169.

116. Tatton NA. Increased caspase 3 and Bax immunoreactivity accompany nuclear GAPDH translocation and neuronal apoptosis in Parkinson's disease. Exp Neurol 2000;166:29.

117. Hartmann A, Troadec JD, Hunot S, et al. Caspase-8 is an effector in apoptotic death of dopaminergic neurons in Parkinson's disease, but pathway inhibition results in neuronal necrosis. J Neurosci 2001;21:2247.

118. Blandini F, Cosentino M, Mangiagalli A, et al. Modifications of apoptosis-related protein levels in lymphocytes of patients with Parkinson's disease. The effect of dopaminergic treatment. J Neural Transm 2004;111:1017.

119. The Parkinson Study Group PRECEPT Investigators. Mixed lineage kinase inhibitor CEP-1347 fails to delay disability in early Parkinson disease. Neurology 2007;69:1480.

120. Andringa G, van Oosten RV, Unger W, et al. Systemic administration of the propargylamine CGP 3466B prevents behavioural and morphological deficits in rats with 6-hydroxydopamine-induced lesions in the substantia nigra. Eur J Neurosci 2000;12:3033.

121. Olanow CW, Schapira AH, LeWitt PA, et al. TCH346 as a neuroprotective drug in Parkinson's disease: a double-blind, randomised, controlled trial. Lancet Neurol 2006;5:1013.

122. Yang L, Sugama S, Mischak RP, et al. A novel systemically active caspase inhibitor attenuates the toxicities of MPTP, malonate, and 3NP in vivo. Neurobiol Dis 2004;17:250.

123. Schierle GS, Hansson O, Leist M, et al. Caspase inhibition reduces apoptosis and increases survival of nigral transplants. Nat Med 1999;5:97.
124. Olanow CW. Rationale for considering that propargylamines might be neuroprotective in Parkinson's disease. Neurology 2006;66:S69.
125. Bonuccelli U, Del Dotto P. New pharmacologic horizons in the treatment of Parkinson disease. Neurology 2006;67:S30.
126. Maruyama W, Nitta A, Shamoto-Nagai M, et al. N-Propargyl-1 (R)-aminoindan, rasagiline, increases glial cell line-derived neurotrophic factor (GDNF) in neuroblastoma SH-SY5Y cells through activation of NF-kappaB transcription factor. Neurochem Int 2004;44:393.
127. de la Lastra CA, Villegas I, Sanchez-Fidalgo S. Poly(ADP-ribose) polymerase inhibitors: new pharmacological functions and potential clinical implications. Curr Pharm Des 2007;13:933.
128. Peng QL, Buz'Zard AR, Lau BH. Pycnogenol protects neurons from amyloid-beta peptide-induced apoptosis. Brain Res Mol Brain Res 2002;104:55.
129. Gutekunst CA, Norflus F, Hersch SM. Recent advances in Huntington's disease. Curr Opin Neurol 2000;13:445.
130. Vis JC, Schipper E, de Boer-van Huizen RT, et al. Expression pattern of apoptosis-related markers in Huntington's disease. Acta Neuropathol 2005; 109:321.
131. Correia SC, Moreira PI. Hypoxia-inducible factor 1: a new hope to counteract neurodegeneration? J Neurochem 2009. [Epub ahead of print].
132. Diaz-Hernandez M, Diez-Zaera M, Sanchez-Nogueiro J, et al. Altered P2X7-receptor level and function in mouse models of Huntington's disease and therapeutic efficacy of antagonist administration. FASEB J 2009;23:1893.
133. Ferrer I, Planas AM. Signaling of cell death and cell survival following focal cerebral ischemia: life and death struggle in the penumbra. J Neuropathol Exp Neurol 2003;62:329.
134. Yang Y, Candelario-Jalil E, Thompson JF, et al. Increased intranuclear matrix metalloproteinase activity in neurons interferes with oxidative DNA repair in focal cerebral ischemia. J Neurochem 2009. [Epub ahead of print].
135. Wu TW, Li WW, Li H. Netrin-1 attenuates ischemic stroke-induced apoptosis. Neuroscience 2008;156:475.
136. Jia J, Guan D, Zhu W, et al. Estrogen inhibits fas-mediated apoptosis in experimental stroke. Exp Neurol 2009;215:48.
137. Abeliovich A, Schmitz Y, Farinas I, et al. Mice lacking alpha-synuclein display functional deficits in the nigrostriatal dopamine system. Neuron 2000;25:239.
138. Lo Bianco C, Schneider B, Bauer M, et al. Lentiviral vector delivery of parkin prevents dopaminergic degeneration in an α-synuclein rat model of Parkinson's disease. Proc Natl Acad Sci 2004;101(50):17510.
139. Kramer ML, Schulz-Schaeffer WJ. Presynaptic alpha-synuclein aggregates, not Lewy bodies, cause neurodegeneration in dementia with Lewy bodies. J Neurosci 2007;27:1405.
140. Bieler S, Soto C. Beta-sheet breakers for Alzheimer's disease therapy. Curr Drug Targets 2004;5:553.
141. Hughes E, Burke RM, Doig AJ. Inhibition of toxicity in the beta-amyloid peptide fragment beta -(25-35) using N-methylated derivatives: a general strategy to prevent amyloid formation. J Biol Chem 2000;275:25109.
142. Bodles AM, El-Agnaf OM, Greer B, et al. Inhibition of fibril formation and toxicity of a fragment of alpha-synuclein by an N-methylated peptide analogue. Neurosci Lett 2004;359:89.

143. Paleologou KE, Irvine GB, El-Agnaf OM. Alpha-synuclein aggregation in neurodegenerative diseases and its inhibition as a potential therapeutic strategy. Biochem Soc Trans 2005;33:1106.

144. El-Agnaf OM, Paleologou KE, Greer B, et al. A strategy for designing inhibitors of alpha-synuclein aggregation and toxicity as a novel treatment for Parkinson's disease and related disorders. FASEB J 2004;18:1315.

145. Masliah E, Hashimoto M. Development of new treatments for Parkinson's disease in transgenic animal models: a role for beta-synuclein. Neurotoxicology 2002;23:461.

146. Rochet JC, Conway KA, Lansbury PT Jr. Inhibition of fibrillization and accumulation of prefibrillar oligomers in mixtures of human and mouse alpha-synuclein. Biochemistry 2000;39:10619.

147. Galvin JE. Interaction of alpha-synuclein and dopamine metabolites in the pathogenesis of Parkinson's disease: a case for the selective vulnerability of the substantia nigra. Acta Neuropathol 2006;112:115.

148. Amijee H, Madine J, Middleton DA, et al. Inhibitors of protein aggregation and toxicity. Biochem Soc Trans 2009;37:692.

149. Brunden KR, Trojanowski JQ, Lee VM. Advances in tau-focused drug discovery for Alzheimer's disease and related tauopathies. Nat Rev Drug Discov 2009;8:783.

150. Nagai Y, Popiel HA. Conformational changes and aggregation of expanded polyglutamine proteins as therapeutic targets of the polyglutamine diseases: exposed beta-sheet hypothesis. Curr Pharm Des 2008;14:3267.

151. Gill SS, Patel NK, Hotton GR, et al. Direct brain infusion of glial cell line-derived neurotrophic factor in Parkinson disease. Nat Med 2003;9:589.

152. Peterson AL, Nutt JG. Treatment of Parkinson's disease with trophic factors. Neurotherapeutics 2008;5:270.

153. Bensadoun JC, Deglon N, Tseng JL, et al. Lentiviral vectors as a gene delivery system in the mouse midbrain: cellular and behavioral improvements in a 6-OHDA model of Parkinson's disease using GDNF. Exp Neurol 2000;164:15.

154. Marshall VL, Grosset DG. GPI-1485 (Guilford). Curr Opin Investig Drugs 2004;5:107.

155. Poulter MO, Payne KB, Steiner JP. Neuroimmunophilins: a novel drug therapy for the reversal of neurodegenerative disease? Neuroscience 2004;128:1.

156. Dass B, Olanow CW, Kordower JH. Gene transfer of trophic factors and stem cell grafting as treatments for Parkinson's disease. Neurology 2006;66:S89.

157. Kompoliti K, Chu Y, Shannon KM, et al. Neuropathological study 16 years after autologous adrenal medullary transplantation in a Parkinson's disease patient. Mov Disord 2007;22:1630.

158. Li JY, Englund E, Holton JL, et al. Lewy bodies in grafted neurons in subjects with Parkinson's disease suggest host-to-graft disease propagation. Nat Med 2008;14:501.

159. Mendez I, Vinuela A, Astradsson A, et al. Dopamine neurons implanted into people with Parkinson's disease survive without pathology for 14 years. Nat Med 2008;14:507.

160. Braak H, Del Tredici K. Assessing fetal nerve cell grafts in Parkinson's disease. Nat Med 2008;14:483.

161. Blurton-Jones M, Kitazawa M, Martinez-Coria H, et al. Neural stem cells improve cognition via BDNF in a transgenic model of Alzheimer disease. Proc Natl Acad Sci U S A 2009;106:13594.

162. Henderson VW. Estrogens, episodic memory, and Alzheimer's disease: a critical update. Semin Reprod Med 2009;27:283.

Healthy Aging Persons and Their Brains: Promoting Resilience Through Creative Engagement

Susan H. McFadden, PhD[a],*, Anne D. Basting, PhD[b]

KEYWORDS

- Creativity • Resilience • Dementia
- Psychosocial interventions • Flourishing

Most older people respond to researchers' questions about their well-being by affirming satisfaction with their lives. They do this despite mounting losses in physical functionality, meaningful social roles and relationships, and the status and respect accorded them by their communities. Called by some "the paradox of well-being,"[1] this resistance to giving in to multiple, objective life challenges has sent researchers looking for other predictors of positive adaption to the exigencies of aging. Borrowing from work with children who thrive despite maltreatment and poverty, women who survive horrific abuse, and military personnel who do not develop posttraumatic stress disorder (PTSD), some researchers, clinicians, and persons who design programs for older adults are beginning to acknowledge older people's resilience, even while they debate how to define and measure it.[2]

The physical sciences describe resilient materials that can return to their original form after being bent, twisted, or stretched. They "bounce back" just as people do when they encounter adversity. One major difference, of course, is that people can learn and grow psychologically and socially in the face of life circumstances that bend, twist, and stretch them[3] and, unlike plastic materials, they are never the same afterwards. The question of what shapes a person's capacity for resilience is now occupying researchers focusing on multiple levels of analysis (biologic, psychosocial, and environmental) that interact dynamically across the life span.[4]

---

[a] Department of Psychology, University of Wisconsin Oshkosh, 800 Algoma Boulevard, Oshkosh, WI 54901, USA
[b] Center on Age and Community, University of Wisconsin Milwaukee, PO Box 413, Milwaukee, WI 53201-0413, USA
* Corresponding author.
E-mail address: mcfadden@uwosh.edu (S.H. McFadden).

Clin Geriatr Med 26 (2010) 149–161
doi:10.1016/j.cger.2009.11.004
0749-0690/10/$ – see front matter © 2010 Elsevier Inc. All rights reserved.

In contradiction to the paradox of well-being observed so often in older adults, elders are often stereotyped as being inflexible and rigid, even though it is less likely that they could have reached late life if they had not been able to respond adaptively to life's challenges.[5] A related stereotype attached to aging people, especially those with the progressive forgetfulness of dementia, is of a passive, downward slide into oblivion. Rarely are persons living with dementia described as having a bounce-back capacity. Instead, they are portrayed as having "ill-being," aging unsuccessfully, and being incapable of experiencing satisfaction with their lives. Some persons diagnosed with Alzheimer disease and other forms of dementia do reflect these stereotypes, but the authors agree with Kitwood[6] and others who argue that this bleak portrayal reflects not the pathology of the brain but the person's response to a malignant social environment.

With supportive social networks and community resources, people with dementia can show a variety of coping strategies, positive emotions, acceptance of their changing situation, and a sense of life meaning.[7] Engaging in creative activities (eg, storytelling, painting, songwriting, dance, and drama) enables people with memory loss to express their strengths. These activities not only reflect resilience; they may also reinforce it biologically, psychologically, and socially.

Although research on the outcomes of older adults' creative engagement is just beginning, some early findings point to its association with physical and mental health. Cohen and colleagues[8] conducted a multisite study with older people (mean age of 80 years) randomly assigned to intervention groups that engaged in some kind of participatory arts activity or control groups that maintained their usual activities. Data from one phase of the study (featuring a musical chorale in Washington, DC) have been published. They show that the intervention group had significantly fewer doctor visits, less medication use, fewer falls, better morale, less loneliness, and higher levels of activity.[8] Cohen suggests that these findings result from participants feeling a greater sense of control and mastery in their lives, and having meaningful and stimulating social engagement.[9] A smaller, short-term intervention study with partial random assignment of community-dwelling elders to a theater group, visual arts group, and a control group that had no intervention, found that theater participants (who had to memorize lines from plays) showed significant improvement on tests of recall and problem solving, and an increase in psychological well-being.[10] The authors of this study attributed the results to the combination of intellectual and social stimulation provided by the theater training.

The following sections draw connections between resilience and creative engagement, arguing that people demonstrate resilience through their acts of creativity. In addition, the opportunity to express oneself through creativity can promote a sense of control and strengthen social ties, thus supporting resilience. Although there are many intersecting pathways to resilience, laid down over the course of life, some of which are less mutable than others (eg, genotypes), nevertheless the authors believe that observations about resilience and creativity lead to intriguing suggestions about future directions for research, clinical practice, and public policy aimed at supporting late-life meaning and purpose, and possibly even slowing the effects of cognitive aging. Evidence is cited suggesting that creative engagement, as an expression of and a support for resilience, may have a neuroprotective effect, contributing to retention of cognitive capacity. Our argument for this hinges on 2 assumptions: that the brain is a social organ,[11] and that resilience and creative engagement are nurtured best in supportive, accepting communities.

CREATIVITY, RESILIENCE, AND AGING: LEO AND MRS G

The term *creative engagement* covers a wide array of activities that extend beyond, but include, the arts. People display creativity when they bring something new that has value into the world.[12] Some differentiate "big C" creativity (meaning the work of professional artists, writers, musicians, playwrights, and others) from the "little c" creativity of ordinary people whose new and valuable productions can include a poem written for a grandchild's birthday, a recipe modified to take advantage of garden vegetables, a song written in celebration of a friend's retirement, or a story told by a campfire. Creative engagement differs from the activities that take place in art, music, and dance therapy because its goal is not the amelioration of psychological or physical symptoms and it does not rely on the participation of a professional therapist. The primary goals of intentional creative engagement programs designed for older persons are to encourage individual expression and to strengthen social connections.

Some older persons involved in creative engagement programs comfortably describe themselves as artists, usually because they have had arts training and have self-identified as artists throughout their lives. Others, in the same programs, refuse the label of "artist." Nevertheless, regardless of whether they call themselves artists, their work activates the same cognitive processes. Lindauer,[13] who extensively studied late-life creativity, described these processes as follows:

> Both nonartists and artists try to figure out what a work might or should mean: they interpret, judge, imagine, evaluate, and make decisions. With few or no clear guidelines, both nonartists and artists search their memories, associations, ideas, and other mental resources; reflexive, routine or habitual responses will not do. Artists and nonartists purposefully search for relevant connections, discard extraneous paths, and organize what remains. (p. 21).

Cognitive psychologists Bink and Marsh[14] observe that the same processes of everyday cognition are used by all people engaged in creative activities, regardless of the individual variations in their outcomes. These include "working memory capacity, speed of retrieval, perceptual fluency, activation of relevant conceptions and inhibition of irrelevant ones, recollective ability, inspection of memories" (p. 75) and many other components of cognition. Given the accumulating research on the enrichment effects of intellectual stimulation for older adults,[15] along with studies showing the connection between social interaction and preservation of cognitive functioning,[15–21] it is possible to understand the growing interest in creative engagement among researchers, practitioners, and persons who develop public policy affecting research on aging and provision of senior services.

Creativity emerges early in childhood[22] and develops across the lifespan. Later life offers many people the opportunity to put aside the demands of work that may have stifled creativity earlier in life.[12] Today, senior centers, community colleges, and universities offer classes designed for older adults who want to learn to paint, compose music, make pottery, write fiction, and explore many other forms of creative expression. Because there are no entry requirements for these courses other than the ability to pay for them, undoubtedly they enroll people who have diagnosed or undiagnosed early memory loss. In addition, a wide variety of programs that encourage creative engagement by persons living with dementia are being introduced into adult day services and long-term care residences.[23] Memories in the Making, a painting program that is supported by the Alzheimer's Association, along with the TimeSlips creative storytelling method, which has been adopted by many organizations serving persons with dementia, are but 2 examples. Individuals who have lost the ability to communicate verbally can find new ways of expressing themselves through these and other creative engagement activities.

The connection between creative engagement and older people's resilience in the face of multiple life challenges has not been directly studied. Bonnano,[24] a leading researcher on resilience, has suggested that creative activities demonstrate people's "capacity for positive emotions and generative experiences" (p. 136) following loss and trauma, but, to our knowledge, no direct links have been studied empirically. Thus, it is necessary to triangulate the evidence to uncover connections between creativity and the psychosocial components of resilience.

One of the earliest studies on resilience in older adults reported on a 10-year follow-up of a national sample of more than 14,000 married and widowed persons. Results showed little or no difference in measures of mortality, self-rated health, activities of daily living, social network size, psychological well-being, depression, and the personality traits of extraversion and openness to experience.[25] The only differences identified were described in terms of lifestyle changes (p. 133): widowed persons had lower income and (in the terminology of the 1980s), were "more likely to have been institutionalized" (p. 129)[25] with 10.8% of the widowed persons living in nursing homes or other institutions compared with 3% of those who were still married at the time of the follow-up. McCrae and Costa[25] concluded that, overall, the widowed elders in their sample experienced no long-term effects on psychosocial functioning. Indeed, they stated that "the great majority of individuals show considerable ability to adapt to a major life stress and continuing life strains—an ability we would call remarkable if it were not so nearly universal a process" (p. 138).[25]

There is no way of knowing whether the persons who participated in McCrae and Costa's research were in any way involved with creative activities. Did they knit sweaters or carve toys for grandchildren, sing in their church choir, paint, write poetry, or compose songs? Other studies of resilience might suggest that they probably recognized that they could not control all aspects of their lives, had a sense of humor, felt committed to important persons and ideas, believed in their ability to manage life, and had close, positive relationships with other people. These are a few of the characteristics of resilient people cited in the literature reviewed by Connor and Davidson,[26] developers of a 25-item validated scale of resilience. As noted by Lindauer,[13] people performing creative activities work toward a goal, feel a sense of purpose, do not give in to discouragement over failure, and feel proud of their achievements; all attributes of resilience cited by Connor and Davidson.

Connor and Davidson's[26] instrument to measure resilience was developed with the participation of middle-aged persons in the general public, psychiatric outpatients, and persons enrolled in studies of generalized anxiety disorder and PTSD. Presumably, all could read and respond to items requiring them to reflect on feelings experienced during the previous month. Leo, and many people like him, would not be able to do this.

Leo has lived in a county-run nursing home for several years. His dementia has progressed to the point at which he utters few words. Nevertheless, Leo was selected to participate in an artist-led program that enabled a group of about 10 residents to make and paint clay pots, take photographs using Polaroid cameras, paint on canvas, draw with colored pencils, assemble a mosaic, and do the preparatory work that resulted in brightly colored fused glass objects. Each time the group met, someone pushed Leo's wheelchair into the room and up to the table holding the art. Leo soon showed his capacity for concentration and meticulous attention to detail. For example, when working with mosaics, he used a small paintbrush to swab on the glue, and then turned it around so he could use the other end to push the mosaic piece into position. Occasionally, he looked up from his work and smiled at the group. About halfway through the 10-week program, the person in charge of activities at the facility commented that Leo was starting to look forward to the arts group. She inferred this from his facial expressions when she said things like "tomorrow the arts group meets." Also around this time, Leo's wife died. He missed a couple of arts group gatherings and the staff respected his wishes not to participate. He returned on the day of the glass-fusing project, and again showed intense concentration, carefully working with his pieces of glass.

Is Leo resilient? This can only be known by observing him, for he is not capable of completing a survey or responding to interview question like the ones Harris posed in her research on resilience in persons with dementia. Harris's[7] assertion that the notion of "successful aging" needs to be replaced with a focus on resilience was based on interviews with persons living with the early stages of memory loss; people who could answer her questions like Mrs G did:

I'm very productive at the moment, so I am going with it. I do [silk] flower floral arrangements for weddings. I am very creative. With silk flowers, I can always have them on hand and keep a prototype. I keep it so I can refer to it because I won't be able to remember how I did that. These things come from my mind. It's my creation. (p. 56)

Leo and Mrs G exercised control through their creative activities; activities that also strengthened their connections to others. Leo knew just where he wanted to place the mosaic and glass pieces; Mrs G had control over the silk flower arrangements. Leo's creativity occurred in a group setting, and required the support and guidance of an artist, volunteers, and staff members. At the end of each session, each person showed what had been made and received applause and cheers from the others. Mrs G made her flower arrangements for the happy occasions of weddings and presumably she got satisfaction from their appreciation of her work.

Researchers studying creative engagement by older persons (including those like Leo and Mrs G who are living with dementia) would be well advised to take seriously the critique offered by Ryff and colleagues[5] regarding research on late-life resilience. They noted the limited perspective in many investigations that operationalize evidence of resilience as the absence of physical and mental illness. Avoiding psychopathology and negative behaviors are "the usual gold standards" (p. 72) defining late-life resilience. Similarly, late-life creativity is beginning to be described in terms of its role in slowing brain aging and avoiding the neuropathology of dementia. As an alternative, Ryff and colleagues propose an emphasis on people's ability to thrive and flourish, which opens up a different way of thinking about creative engagement and resilience. The authors do not deny that encouragement of resilience and support for creative engagement can produce positive outcomes for health. The challenge lies in maintaining a multiple levels of analysis approach that does not reduce human complexity to mechanisms of brain function.[4,15]

Another perspectival shift that is important for considering creativity, resilience, and aging relates to fundamental assumptions about selfhood. Selfhood is relational. That is, people's sense of who they are, and their capacity to adapt to internal and external challenges across the lifespan, are formed in relationship with other persons.[27] Although cultural stereotypes envision creative people working alone, creativity and the arts are fundamentally social, for the product of creative endeavor is nearly always shared with others. Likewise, despite the stereotypical equation of resilience with rugged individualism, people's resilience is expressed and supported in a social context.

WHAT'S GOOD FOR THE PERSON IS USUALLY GOOD FOR THE BRAIN

A growing body of scientific evidence affirms the connection between meaningful relationships in a diverse social network and less cognitive decline in old age, greater resistance to infection, and better prognoses in the face of life-threatening illnesses.[28] Nevertheless, despite considerable research effort in the last 2 decades, our understanding of the physiologic mechanisms that produce these results is still fragile and incomplete.[15]

In a report on their own longitudinal study of a community-based sample of elders, and a review of other longitudinal studies examining the benefits of active, socially engaged lives, Fratiglioni and colleagues[29,30] conclude that there is good evidence for a protective effect against dementia when people have rich social networks and engage in various mental and physical activities. Their lifespan model is multidimensional; it includes risk factors (genetics, poverty, depression, hypertension and other vascular problems, and head trauma) and additional protective factors such as education, good diet, and control of hypertension and cholesterol. Other studies affirm the findings of Fratiglioni and colleagues: older persons who have higher levels of social engagement experience less cognitive decline,[15–21] along with a greater sense of life meaning and purpose,[31] and more likelihood that they will flourish as they cope with late-life challenges.[32,33]

None of these studies specifically examined creative engagement, but in their lists of various types of activities that older people may do together, one finds several that express creativity. For example, in 2 prospective studies showing that leisure activities reduce the risk of dementia and of amnestic mild cognitive impairment, Verghese and colleagues[34,35] included playing musical instruments and dancing. In addition to not noting the creative element in certain social activities, these studies did not include measures of resilience. However, when one compares the biopsychosocial mechanisms they cite as protective against cognitive decline and those other researchers cite as reflecting resilience, one finds similar factors at work. This finding is most plainly seen in studies of allostasis and allostatic load.

Allostasis refers to the way organisms maintain stability in the midst of change; it reflects an internal balancing mechanism that responds and adapts to external demands through the coordinated functioning of the neuroendocrine system, the immune system, and the autonomic nervous system.[36] Allostatic load describes "strain on multiple organs and tissues that accumulates via the wear and tear associated with *acute shifts* in physiologic reactivity in response to negative stimuli and via *chronic elevations* in physiologic activity."[5] It is the physiologic cost of problematic management of stress which produces the cumulative effect of wear and tear on the body, including, of course, the brain. However, this is not the whole story, for biologic and psychological resilience can offset these allostatic demands. Optimal allostasis (and reduction of allostatic load) occurs via 2 pathways that have physiologic sequelae: "effective warding off of stress" and "encounters with the positives of life."[5] Maintaining meaningful social relationships and engaging in mentally stimulating generative activities are 2 ways of doing this, and, of course, they often co-occur.

Have Leo and Mrs G experienced allostatic load? It is associated with conditions like hypertension, suppression of the immune system, hippocampal atrophy, and memory impairment.[36] Given that Leo and Mrs G have been diagnosed with dementia, it is likely that their brains and vascular systems show the cumulative effects of meeting the challenges of human life. Does this mean they failed at aging, that instead of aging well they are aging ill? Using McCrae and Costa's[25] terminology of the 1980s, Leo has been institutionalized. He needs considerable assistance from others for most activities of daily life. As reported by Harris,[7] Mrs G has "very bad asthma and emphysema and a few years earlier had cancer surgery" (p. 3). She was forced to retire early because of the dementia diagnosis, and she gets little help from her sons and 12 siblings. On the other hand, Leo lives in a progressive facility dedicated to supporting personhood in all residents and Mrs G has a loving husband, a support network in her community, and an understanding physician. Within the constraints of their lives, both show resilience. One might even say that, within these constraints, they are flourishing and their creative expressions are but one example of the lived experience of the paradox of well-being.

IMPLICATIONS FOR RESEARCH, PRACTICE, AND POLICY

Because of the ferment over support for the arts in children's education in recent years, more research on creativity and cognitive capacity has focused on the early years than the later years of life. Those who study older people would be well advised to become more familiar with this literature. Since the early 1990s, cognitive neuroscientists have been attempting to understand why arts training for children seems to be associated with better academic performance. This research suggests that training in arts performance (especially music, theater, and dance) produces high states of motivation, which in turn enable greater attention and affect children's memory and cognition.[37,38]

This literature holds promise for researchers who study people at the other end of the life span. For example, "motivational reserve" (which reflects activities like planning, goal-setting, and feelings that one is capable of accomplishing a task) has been suggested as yet another protective factor against late-life cognitive impairment.[39] Leo and Mrs G showed various aspects of motivation in their creative activities. Researchers should consider whether activating motivational reserve through creative engagement can slow the progress of cognitive decline. Studies of the role of sustained attention in the relationship between arts training and children's cognition remind us of Leo's focus on the mosaics and glass pieces, and Mrs G's attention to detail in her silk flower arrangements. People who are unfamiliar with creative engagement programs for persons with dementia are often surprised at their ability to maintain attention for as long as an hour or more. Is this attention offering them protection against further cognitive decline? No research has yet addressed this question. Observe children learning their lines for a play, community-dwelling older people planning a musical performance, or people with dementia creating a story together and you will see determination to reach a goal, focused attention, and, usually, a lot of smiles and laughter. Although far more is known about how negative emotions affect health than is known about positive emotions, some empirical evidence is beginning to show that good feelings have salutary outcomes, producing greater resilience, better immune system function, and less inflammation,[40] all of which would benefit vascular and brain health.

Given all this, the authors suggest that researchers interested in the outcomes of older persons' creative engagement activities account for their motivational, attentional, affective, and social attributes, and their cognitive components, realizing, of course, the complex reciprocal interactions among these phenomena. Creative engagement research must maintain a multiple levels of analysis approach like that

Table 1
Creative engagement programs and resources

Program Name and Description	Resources and Contact Information
ArtCare Located at Luther Manor Adult Day Services in Milwaukee, WI, this program offers annual artist residencies. Artists work with staff and day center participants for 15 weeks, culminating with a public display of the art	http://www.luthermanor.org ArtCare Manual (written by Anne Basting) This gives step-by-step instructions on how to incorporate an arts program into long-term care. It can be ordered from the Center on Age and Community: http://www.aging.uwm.edu
Artists for Alzheimers (ARTZ) This nonprofit organization trains artists to volunteer with persons with dementia. It is based at Hearthstone Alzheimer's Care	http://www.artistsforalzheimers.org
Arts for the Aging (AFTA) Artists in the Washington, DC, area provide programs to senior organizations working with underserved elders	http://www.aftaarts.org
Center for Elders and Youth in the Arts (CEYA) Based in San Francisco, this organization connects elders and youth in arts programming	http://ceya.ioaging.org
DanceWorks Artists offer dance workshops in Milwaukee area adult day centers	http://www.danceworksmke.org
Duplex Planet Founder David Greenberger conducts unconventional interviews with elders and transforms them into art forms such as songs and graphic novels	http://www.duplexplanet.com
Elders Share the Arts (ESTA) Programs in New York City use visual arts and storytelling with older people	http://www.eldersharethearts.org Several training manuals are available from ESTA
Kairos Dance Theater An intergenerational dance company, Kairos Dance Theater provides staff training in dance for elders with dementia through The Dancing Heart program	http://www.kairosdance.org
Liz Lerman Dance Exchange Dance workshops and performances for elders, including those with dementia	http://www.danceexchange.org Offers a free, online "toolbox" with exercises designed to elicit creativity

Memories in the Making Art program involving painting, adopted by many Alzheimer's Association chapters	http://www.alz.org/oc/in_my_community_10849.asp Staff trainings are offered; a training manual and DVD are also available
Next Stage Dance Theater (NSDT) Dance programs for persons with dementia living in the Seattle area	http://www.nextstagedance.org
Opening Minds Through Art (OMA) A service-learning arts program in which students create art with older adults with dementia. Based in Ohio	http://www.omaproject.org
Songwriting Works Offers staff training in group songwriting for persons living with dementia	http://www.songwritingworks.org
StoryCorps National oral history project enabling families and friends to record people's stories of their lives. The Memory Loss Initiative focuses on persons with dementia	http://www.storycorps.net
TimeSlips Group storytelling process created by Anne Basting. Training and consultation offered through the Center on Age and Community in Milwaukee, WI	http://www.timeslips.org Training manual, DVD, and images for storytelling are available through the Web site
Transitional Keys Offers tools to provide meaning and fulfillment at times of change and transition, especially those marked by celebrations, losses, and major turning points	http://www.transitionalkeys.org

Data from Basting AD. Forget memory: creating better lives for people with dementia. Baltimore, MD: The Johns Hopkins University Press; 2009. This book includes detailed descriptions of these and other related programs.

emphasized by scientists studying resilience[4] and preservation and enhancement of older adults' cognitive capacity.[15]

Although brain health is the goal of some people who promote creative engagement as an intervention, the authors believe the emphasis needs to be expanded to include goals of improving psychological well-being, nurturing social relationships, and supporting a sense of life meaning and purpose, all of which undergird resilience. As noted by Manepalli and colleagues,[41] psychosocial approaches like creative engagement programs support resilience by increasing a sense of mastery and control, along with strengthening social connections. These approaches benefit persons with conditions like Alzheimer disease, their family members, and other care partners.

The authors observed this among participants in a "brain and memory fitness program" sponsored by a geriatric psychiatry clinic called the Alzheimer's Center of Excellence, located in Appleton, WI. A group of about 10 persons diagnosed with early stage dementia met regularly with a nurse and a geriatric nurse practitioner at the same clinic where they also had appointments with their geriatric psychiatrist and had gone through extensive neuropsychological testing. Often, people enter a medical office looking serious, even worried, about what might transpire there. In contrast, the participants in this group greeted one another happily as they walked from the parking lot into the building, anticipating the 90 minutes they would spend together in a program that included meditation, a creative activity, informal conversation, and structured discussion. Together, they designed a poster featuring what they named the "sun of mindfulness," a bright orange figure with the words "peace, love, and joy." On the poster (later reproduced and laminated as an 8.5 in by 11 in sign, and a smaller calling card), they listed creative, stillness, relational, spiritual, imagery, and movement practices that they believed would give them a sense of peace, love, and joy. What a different message this provides from the usual grim statistics about aging and cognitive decline, conversion from mild cognitive impairment to Alzheimer disease, and the emotional and financial costs of dementia care.

The authors have no data on whether the individuals in this group would score higher on measures of resilience or cognitive capacity than a matched control group in a randomized trial. However, given the triangulation of evidence that is presented here, the authors believe there is sufficient reason to encourage clinicians to alert older persons, regardless of their cognitive status, to the positive benefits of getting together with others to enjoy creative activities (**Table 1** shows examples of creative engagement programs and resources). As noted by Manepalli and colleagues,[41] pharmacotherapy for many of the behavioral and emotional concomitants of dementia can be ineffective and even risky. The current medical paradigm that devalues psychosocial interventions by calling them "nonpharmacologic" needs to be replaced with one that recognizes that "a relationship *is* a physiologic process, as real and as potent as any pill or surgical procedure."[42]

These recommendations have implications for policy makers and clinicians. Policy makers influence the distribution of research dollars. The current focus on finding biomedical cures and treatments for the cognitive changes wrought by aging often seems blind to the social nature of human life. Funding for research on psychosocial approaches to improving the well-being of older people is miniscule compared with biomedical research, and yet it exists on just as solid a scientific base, testing theories with good design, valid and reliable measures, and caution about effect sizes.

Over the years, the United States has developed policies about drug advertising. Similar policies now need to be developed about activities that fall into the general category of "brain training" for aging persons. Research on such cognitive interventions for healthy aging people gets distorted in the popular press, preventing the public from making good decisions about investing their time and money in such programs, many of which fail to demonstrate any significant effects in preventing or slowing cognitive decline.[43] The authors can foresee unsubstantiated dose response claims being made about creative activities (eg, paint using our system for 30 minutes a day and experience improved memory and resilience in 1 month) just as similar claims are now being made about various technologies that supposedly promote "brain fitness." These will require close regulatory scrutiny.

Although there continue to be gaps and weaknesses in research on creativity and resilience, there is enough evidence about the biopsychological benefits of social engagement to promote policies supporting programs that enable older people to gather with others to express themselves through creative activities of all kinds. Coalitions of persons involved with the arts and advocates for elders, including persons living with dementia, need to strategize on raising awareness among voters and politicians about the benefits of providing creative engagement activities in venues including public libraries, colleges, and skilled nursing residences. In addition to the positive outcomes accruing to participants in these activities, greater community awareness of creative productions by older people could reduce the stigma associated with aging and dementia and broaden public images of life in old age beyond the usual lists of mental and physical disorders.[44]

SUMMARY OF KEY POINTS

Will creative engagement preserve brain function and prevent dementia? Research points toward this possibility for some, but certainly not all, persons. As Hertzog and colleagues[15] comment at the end of their review of research on cognitive enrichment, "even individuals who engage in optimal enrichment behaviors will probably experience adverse cognitive changes at some point in the end-game of life" (p. 49). Thus, this discussion turns eventually toward enduring existential and spiritual questions about life meaning and its roots in individual lives and in community. Communities of persons who understand that joys and sorrows intermingle in a long life might better grasp a vision of older adult well-being as not so paradoxic after all.

There is much that is still not known about the multiple, dynamically interacting influences on cognitive aging that begin with conception. Nevertheless, there is now evidence about the psychosocial benefits of creative activities; activities that express and uphold elders' resilience regardless of their cognitive status. These activities, engaged in by imaginative human beings sharing their work with others, can elicit joy, promote life meaning, and strengthen the bonds of community that will nurture future generations.

ACKNOWLEDGMENTS

The authors gratefully acknowledge Benjamin Mullins, University of Wisconsin Oshkosh, for his help with the references.

REFERENCES

1. Mroczek DK, Kolarz CM. The effect of age on positive and negative affect: a developmental perspective on happiness. J Pers Soc Psychol 1998;75: 1333–49.
2. Luthar SS, Cicchetti D, Becker B. The construct of resilience: a critical evaluation and guidelines for future work. Child Dev 2000;71:543–62.

3. Park CL, Fenster JR. Stress-related growth: predictors of occurrence and correlates with psychological adjustment. J Soc Clin Psychol 2004;23:195–215.
4. Cicchetti D, Blender JA. A multiple-levels-of-analysis perspective on resilience: implications for the developing brain, neural plasticity, and preventive interventions. Ann N Y Acad Sci 2006;1094:248–58.
5. Ryff CD, Singer B, Love GD, et al. Resilience in adulthood and later life: defining features and dynamic processes. In: Lomranz J, editor. Handbook of aging and mental health: an integrative approach. New York: Plenum Press; 1998. p. 69–96.
6. Kitwood T. Dementia reconsidered: the person comes first. Philadelphia: Open University Press; 1997.
7. Harris PB. Another wrinkle in the debate about successful aging: the undervalued concept of resilience and the lived experience of dementia. Int J Aging Hum Dev 2008;67:43–61.
8. Cohen GD, Perlstein S, Chapline J, et al. The impact of professionally conducted cultural programs on the physical health, mental health, and social functioning of older adults. Gerontologist 2006;46(6):726–34.
9. Cohen GD. Research on creativity and aging: the positive impact of the arts on health and illness. Generations 2006;30(1):7–15.
10. Noice H, Noice T, Staines G. A short-term intervention to enhance cognitive and affective functioning in older adults. J Aging Health 2004;16:562–85.
11. Cozolino L. The healthy aging brain: sustaining attachment, attaining wisdom. New York: W.W. Norton; 2008.
12. Cohen CD. The creative age: awakening human potential in the second half of life. New York: HarperCollins; 2000.
13. Lindauer MS. Aging, creativity, and art: a positive perspective on late-life development. New York: Kluwer Academic/Plenum Publishers; 2003.
14. Bink ML, Marsh RL. Cognitive regularities in creative activity. Rev Gen Psychol 2000;4:59–78.
15. Hertzog C, Kramer AF, Wilson RS, et al. Enrichment effects on adult cognitive development: can the functional capacity of older adults be preserved and enhanced? Psychol Sci 2008;9:1–65.
16. Barnes LL, Mendes de Leon C, Wilson RW, et al. Social resources and cognitive decline in a population of older African Americans and whites. Neurology 2004;63(12):2322–6.
17. Bassuk SS, Glass TA, Berkman LF. Social disengagement and incident cognitive decline in community-dwelling elderly persons. Ann Intern Med 1999;131(3):165–73.
18. Bennett DA, Schneider JA, Tang Y, et al. The effect of social networks on the relation between Alzheimer's disease pathology and level of cognitive function in old people: a longitudinal cohort study. Lancet Neurol 2006;5(5):406–12.
19. Ertel KA, Glymour MM, Berkman LF. Effects of social integration on preserving memory function in a nationally representative US elderly population. Am J Public Health 2008;98(7):1215–20.
20. Glass TA, Mendes de Leon C, Marottoli RA, et al. Population based study of social and productive activities as predictors of survival among elderly Americans. BMJ 1999;319:478–83.
21. Zunzunegui M-V, Alvarado BE, Del Ser T, et al. Social networks, social integration, and social engagement determine cognitive decline in community-dwelling Spanish older adults. J Gerontol B Psychol Sci Soc Sci 2003;58:S93–100.
22. Gardner H. Artful scribbles: the significance of children's drawings. New York: Basic Books; 1980.

23. Basting AD. ArtCare: the story of how an arts program can transform long term care. Milwaukee (WI): UWM Center on Age & Community; 2008.

24. Bonnano GA. Resilience in the face of potential trauma. Curr Dir Psychol Sci 2005;14:135–8.

25. McCrae RR, Costa PT. Psychological resilience among widowed men and women: a 10-year follow-up of a national sample. J Soc Issues 1988;44:129–42.

26. Connor KM, Davidson JRT. Development of a new resilience scale: the Connor-Davidson Resilience Scale (CD-RISC). Depress Anxiety 2003;18(2):76–82.

27. Gergen K. Relational being: beyond self and community. New York: Oxford University Press; 2009.

28. Cohen S, Janicki-Deverts D. Can we improve our physical health by altering our social networks? Perspect Psychol Sci 2009;4(4):375–8.

29. Fratiglioni L, Paillard-Borg S, Winblad B. An active and socially integrated lifestyle in late life might protect against dementia. Lancet Neurol 2004;3:343–53.

30. Fratiglioni L, Wang H-X, Ericsson K, et al. Influence of social network on occurrence of dementia: a community-based longitudinal study. Lancet 2000;355:1315–9.

31. Krause N. Stressors in highly valued roles, meaning in life, and the physical health status of older adults. J Gerontol B Psychol Sci Soc Sci 2004;59:S287–97.

32. Keyes CLM. Chronic physical conditions and aging: is mental health a potential protective factor? Ageing Int 2005;30:88–104.

33. Keyes CLM. Promoting and protecting mental health as flourishing: a complementary strategy for improving national mental health. Am Psychol 2007;62:95–108.

34. Verghese J, LeValley MA, Derby C, et al. Leisure activities and the risk of amnestic mild cognitive impairment in the elderly. Neurology 2006;66:821–7.

35. Verghese J, Lipton RB, Katz MJ, et al. Leisure activities and the risk of dementia in the elderly. N Engl J Med 2003;348:2508–16.

36. McEwen BS. Interacting mediators of allostasis and allostatic load: towards an understanding of resilience in aging. Metabolism 2003;52(10 Suppl 2):10–6.

37. Posner M, Rothbart MK, Sheese BE, et al. How arts training influences cognition. In: Asbury C, Rich B, editors. Learning, arts and the brain. New York: Dana Press; 2004. p. 1–10.

38. Rauscher F, Gruhn W. Neurosciences in music pedagogy. New York: Nova Biomedical Books; 2008.

39. Forstmeier S, Maercker A. Motivational reserve: lifetime motivational abilities contribute to cognitive and emotional health in old age. Psychol Aging 2008;23(4):886–99.

40. Fredrickson BL, Losada MF. Positive affect and the complex dynamics of human flourishing. Am Psychol 2005;60:678–86.

41. Manepalli J, Desai A, Sharma P. Psychosocial-environmental treatments for Alzheimer's disease. Prim Psychiatry 2009;16(6):39–47.

42. Lewis T, Amini R, Lannon R. A general theory of love. New York: Random House; 2000.

43. Papp KV, Walsh SJ, Snyder PJ. Immediate and delayed effects of cognitive interventions in healthy elderly: a review of current literature and future directions. Alzheimers Dement 2009;5:50–60.

44. Basting AD. Forget memory: creating better lives for people with dementia. Baltimore (MD): The Johns Hopkins University Press; 2009.

Index

Note: Page numbers of article titles are in **boldface** type.

A

Academic institutions, role in promotion of healthy brain aging, 11

Advanced Cognitive Training for Independent and Vital Elderly study, 104

Aging persons, activation of motivational reserve in, 155

    allostasis of, 154

    healthy, and their brains, resilience through creative engagement, **149–161**

        creativity, resilience, and aging of, 151–154

    stereotyping of, 150

    things good for, also good for brain, 154–155

Alcohol, and healthy brain aging, 33–36

    beneficial and deleterious effects on brain, 35–36

    chronic consumption of, neuropsychiatric symptoms associated with, 33

    consumption of, Alzheimer disease and, 34

        and dementia, 34, 35

    head injury, and environmental toxins, effect on healthy brain aging, **29–44**

Allostasis, of aging persons, 154

Alzheimer disease, 1, 18

    alcohol consumption and, 34

    apoptosis in, 135

    excitotoxicity and N-methyl-D-aspartate glutamate receptors in, 128–129

    genetic education and counseling on, 8–9

    growth factors and gene therapies in, 139

    hazard ratio of brain injury and, 32

    hypertension as risk factor for, 18

    inactivity and, 75

    inflammation in, 130–131

    intellectual-cultural activities and, 103

    misfolding of protein and protein aggregation in, 137

    mitochondrial dysfunction in, 132–133

    oxidative stress in, 127

    prevention of, physical activity and, epidemiologic studies in, 76–77, 78–79

    risk and protective factors for, 119

    vitamins as benefit in, 127

APOE gene, and risk of dementia following head injury, 32

Apoptosis, in Alzheimer disease, 135

    in Huntington disease, 135

    in Parkinson disease, 134–135

    in stroke, 136

B

Beer, comsumption of, Alzheimer disease and, 35

Benevia, 94

Clin Geriatr Med 26 (2010) 163–170

doi:10.1016/S0749-0690(10)00009-1

geriatric.theclinics.com

0749-0690/10/$ – see front matter © 2010 Elsevier Inc. All rights reserved.

Moving?

Make sure your subscription moves with you!

To notify us of your new address, find your **Clinics Account Number** (located on your mailing label above your name), and contact customer service at:

Email: **journalscustomerservice-usa@elsevier.com**

800-654-2452 (subscribers in the U.S. & Canada)
314-447-8871 (subscribers outside of the U.S. & Canada)

Fax number: **314-447-8029**

Elsevier Health Sciences Division
Subscription Customer Service
3251 Riverport Lane
Maryland Heights, MO 63043

*To ensure uninterrupted delivery of your subscription, please notify us at least 4 weeks in advance of move.

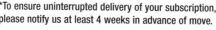